Whis
of H'ope

Dearest Janet

May you always
find peace within.

With Love,
Denise

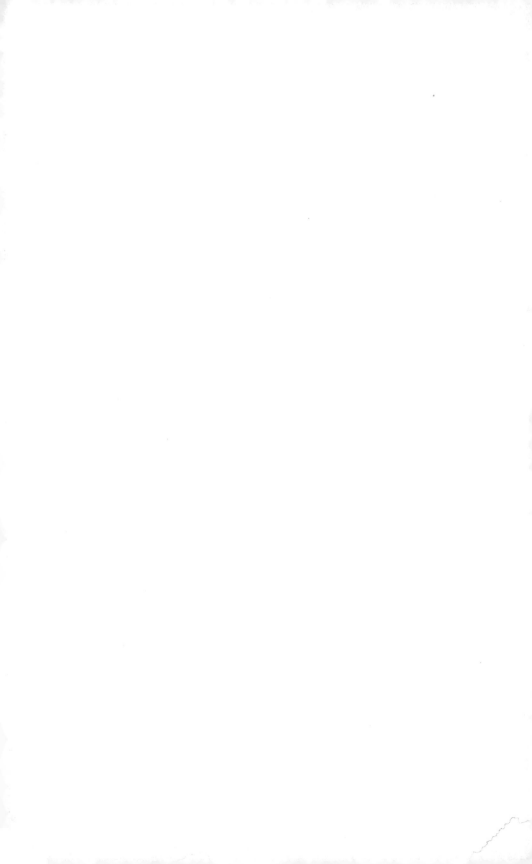

Whispers of Hope

TRANSCENDING ABUSE, CANCER AND DIVORCE TO EMBRACE PEACE

DENISE CUNNINGHAM

Journey Home Publishing Edition, 2011

Cover Photo: © istockphoto.com/wingmar
Author's Photo: Karen Learmonth, Amber Light Photography
Book Design: Joe Gregory. Book Update: Madison Creative Inc.
Lyrics to the song *Lady Lavender* used with kind permission from Sneezer Music © 2010 www.denisehagan.com
First Edition Published in Great Britain

Library and Archives Canada Cataloguing in Publication
Cunningham, Denise Ann, 1959-
    Whispers of hope : transcending abuse, cancer and divorce to embrace peace / Denise Ann Cunningham. -- Rev. ed.

ISBN 978-0-9877135-0-6
    1. Self-actualization (Psychology). 2. Cunningham, Denise Ann, 1959-. 3. Adult child abuse victims--Canada--Biography. 4. Cancer--Patients--Canada--Biography. 5. Counselors--Canada-- Biography. I. Title.

BF637.S4C85 2011   158.1   C2011-907500-8

DISCLAIMER: This book was written from the author's perceptions of events in her life. This may or may not match other's perceptions of the events she describes. Within this work of non-fiction the author has used pseudonyms for her daughters' names to protect their privacy. As well, the author's personal letters within the text have not been edited from their original writing. This self-help guide is intended to offer information of a general nature to help readers in their quest for emotional and spiritual well-being. It is not a replacement for professional health care or mental health advice. Readers may find that some of their past wounds come up to be healed while reading this book. If they feel emotionally overwhelmed at any time they are advised to seek professional support. Readers of this publication agree that neither Denise Ann Cunningham, nor her publisher will be held responsible or liable for damages that may be alleged or resulting, directly, or indirectly, from their use of this publication. All external links are provided as a resource only and are not guaranteed to remain active for any length of time. Neither the publisher nor the author can be held accountable for the information provided by, or actions resulting from accessing these resources.

"When we walk to the edge of all the light we have and take the step into the darkness of the unknown, we must believe that one of two things will happen. There will be something solid for us to stand on or we will be taught to fly."

Patrick Overton

This book is dedicated to the three most important women in my life.

To my mom for being my greatest teacher of compassion and for demonstrating the power of a mother's love in the last years of her life.

And to my beautiful daughters, who are the heart of my soul. It is a gift beyond measure to have you in my life. Thank you for choosing me to be your mother. You continue to teach me how to be a better human being. I love you all ways and forever.

Praise

"*A Course in Miracles* states that a miracle is a shift in perception. *Whispers of Hope* not only shows the miracle of Denise Cunningham's journey from fear to love, it also shows the world how to move from darkness into light. As she changed her past conditioning she transformed her life story into a "Generational Love Story". Denise is a living example of Grace as she embraces the inner core of Dignity we each have within us. As we seek peace in our own hearts, this book is a loving companion on our healing journey. As each of us heals, the ripple effect is felt around the world."

Kim Tebbutt, Reiki Master, Author of *Seven Billion Angels and Counting*

"*Whispers of Hope* is the masterpiece of a quiet, modest hero who survived an unthinkable life. Cunningham's ability to love and rise above time after time after time in her journey reveals her true wisdom as a great teacher for our time. I love this book...it is a powerful, inner trophy for the human spirit."

Denise Hagan, Musician and Song Writer

"Hey Sis, I just read the chapter "Hands". It was so beautifully written and so full of truth it took my breath away. Tears were rolling down my cheeks as I read it. You are a very brave lady to dig into and make sense of all that shit. You tell it exactly as it was. Anyone that has lived through anything like it will feel the truth in those words and maybe won't feel so alone and isolated knowing someone else went through what they did."

Glen Cunningham, Musician and Song Writer

"As a physician, I have come to understand the power of words in the healing process. For those words to have impact, they must be true. They must come from a place, often hard won, of authenticity. The power of *Whispers of Hope* is that it is a book that resonates with honesty. You believe Denise Cunningham and therefore trust her message of hope and the possibility of renewal. This belief and trust in the process outlined in *Whispers of Hope* will be so valuable for anyone travelling the road towards peace and wholeness in their lives."

Nancy Wardle, MD

"*Whispers of Hope* is a wealth of wisdom for all those who are called to personal and collective healing. Denise's story reminds me of an ancient symbol from the East of human life: a beautiful white lotus radiantly blooming up out of the mud. And so it is for each of us. Our very humanity, and all that this entails, is the very ground of our awakening. Denise, as all fine healers do, has risen from the ground of her own very difficult initiation, dared to tell her story, and thus become a guide for the rest of us!"

David Fields, Co-Author of *The Invisible Wedding: Exploring the Essence of Spiritual Partnership*

"Looking at *Whispers of Hope* from my spiritual side, this book is a testament to Denise's ability not to just survive but to learn and evolve from the trials presented to her in her life. She helps guide those of us trying to do the same thing. Looking from the more logical side of me that needs things to be proven to me, Denise offers a number of scientific studies to back up the beliefs she acquired on her own journey and gives a number of practical exercises to help us reach our own beliefs. This makes *Whispers of Hope* a unique contribution to the world of spiritual writing, which sometimes seems rampant with books that have little grounding in the real world, with concepts the average person cannot comprehend. Denise has somehow managed to bring science and spirituality together, succeeding admirably in the process."

Susan McNicoll, Author of *British Columbia Murders*, *Ontario Murders* and *The Opening Act: a biographical history of Canadian theatre from 1945-1953*

"Readers will have many opportunities to relate to Denise's vivid descriptions of her healing journey from childhood trauma to reclaiming her authentic Self. The questions she poses at the end of each chapter offer much food for thought and stimulus to explore further for ourselves. Her honesty in describing her healing process, and where she is now, demonstrates the integrity that is so important to achieving a strong sense of Self and finding peace within. Her wisdom about the role our feelings play in our lives and in our emotional health is invaluable."

Janice Berger, M.Ed., Author of *Emotional Fitness: Discovering Our Natural Healing Power*

"What can be more powerful than what we learn from our own life experience? The question is – do we learn or just experience? Denise does both in this profoundly honest exposition of her life – but more than that, she takes it one step further as she empowers all of us with tools, at the end of each chapter, for our own personal journey of awakening."

Alma Lightbody, Co-Author of *My Wonderful Nightmare*

"*Whispers of Hope* is a gift to humanity. The story is told with the brilliant wisdom of a heart that has lived the loss and disappointment in all of us, and emerged to illuminate our deepest potential to love. It is a heart-breaking and heart-inspiring story of hope -- a guide that gently brings us back to our Highest Self again and again."

Karen McGregor, Bestselling Author of *The Madonna Code: Mysteries of the Divine Feminine Unveiled*

"*Whispers of Hope* is a courageous story of one woman's experience of healing her body of breast cancer. Denise grows beyond the traditional routine of surgery and chemotherapy and takes the path of co-creating health. She inspires all of us to return to the beauty and power of our heart. Denise Cunningham is a very Powerful Woman!"

Nancy Kerner, Creator of Vision Dancer Productions and Author of *The Power of Sexy Relationships*

Contents

Acknowledgements

To my father – Thank you for teaching me about kindness and showing me that life is a gift.

To my brothers Jim and Glen Cunningham – Thank you for 'having my back' always. I love you more than words can say.

To the Uhlmans and the Summerhills – Thank you for believing in me until I learned how to believe in myself.

To my ex-husband – You have seen me at my best and at my worst. Thank you for loving me through it all. You have my eternal gratitude for the gift of our two amazing daughters.

To Donna Brinton, Beth Cook, Fran Ledingham, Judy Dubsky, and my many other beautiful and amazing friends all over the world – I wish I could name every single one of you but that would be another book! Thank you for holding the space for me as I learned how to fly. You have helped to make me who I am.

To my friends, family, co-workers, and caregivers who held the light for me during my cancer diagnosis and treatment – Thank you. Your love made a huge difference.

To Susan McNicoll – my friend and fellow author. Thank you for being my number one fan and for helping me keep my sanity as I ventured into this new arena called 'published writing'! Your unconditional love and support mean more to me than words can say.

To my anam cara Lesley – Thank you for playing Louise to my Thelma. We have supported each other through life after breast cancer and now we get to support each other's dreams. I am grateful to have you in my life.

To the fabulous 5 women from the "Q" – "There you are!" and I am so happy to have found you again in this lifetime. When I am with you I remember the Truth of who I am.

To my clients, past and present, who remind me what an honour and a privilege it is to be invited into another's life – Thank you for your courage and your willingness to trust a complete stranger with your heart.

To my cousin-in-law Robert Kirby: the other writer in the family! – Thank you for taking the time to encourage a budding writer, and for telling me to, "Write what I know."

To all those who supported me through the Next Top Spiritual Author's Contest – we made it into the top 10% of nearly 3,000 writers who entered the competition! Thank you for your consistent reminders that I am a writer.

To my friends at the Divine You Writing Group in White Rock, British Columbia – Thank you for sharing your souls in your writing and for your continued heart-felt support of mine.

To the Spiritual Authors Circle – It has been my great honour to co-create unity consciousness with all of you. You keep me connected to the Divinity within.

To Julie – Thank you for being the mid-wife for my dream.

To my editors and proofreaders – Thank you for catching the glitches and making this book a more polished piece of work.

And lastly, to a beautiful Quarter Horse named Indy and a majestic Friesian named Nyk – Thank you for reminding me what it means to live from my true nature, in the present moment. I promise to hold your message, "You don't have to *do*, just *be*!" in my heart always.

Foreword

"Your task is not to seek love, but merely to seek and find all the barriers within yourself that you have built against it."

Rumi

SOMETIMES YOU DISCOVER A BOOK that resonates with you so deeply you know you will re-read it many times. Throughout my career as a public educator and holistic practitioner, I have read countless books that have led to self-help and personal growth. The ones that resonate with my every vibration, all speak to me with, and bring me back to, the heart connection. Denise Cunningham's *Whispers of Hope: Transcending Abuse, Cancer and Divorce to Embrace Peace* is such a book.

When Denise asked me to write the foreword for this book, a flood of memories came to mind. One of which was our first meeting at a wellness centre where I worked. As we got to know one another over cups of tea, we delved into like-minded discussions. It didn't take long for us to discover that through our many years of self-discovery and transformation, our philosophies of the heart were the same; the belief that we are already perfect and that it is easier to discover that perfection when we are gentle and loving with ourselves.

Denise writes with grace and beauty as her words gently move us through her story. She begins by referring to her past in a fairy tale. By reflecting on abusive childhood incidences in this way she allows herself to be somewhat removed; not to avoid feelings and emotions, but rather to show us, the reader, that she has an awareness she has accumulated through her years of self transformation. An awareness that shows that she can now be the observer, and that what happened in the past doesn't have to affect her present or determine her future. The fairy tale describes her mother's life as well as her own, for our life's experiences begin before our birth. She shares four of the key mistaken beliefs she developed growing up: "Be Quiet, Stop Feeling,

Do Not Ever Fail, and Grow Up – Be An Adult". These were the basis for the many decisions she made throughout the early part of her life.

Whispers of Hope transcends the belief that we all have 'stuff' to work through. It is one woman's story, showing how she began to discover and identify her emotional baggage, and how her perceptions reinforced her mistaken beliefs. We see what we want to see until something happens in our life that wakes us up. Like the unravelling of tapestry threads that have been caught on innocent passers-by, we never know who will catch that thread and run with it. It may be the dog, our partner, a child, or a colleague. The first people to begin this unravelling in Denise were her children. Listening to her inner voice, she allowed herself to be led to those that would help her discover how she got there in the first place. Sometimes quickly, sometimes slowly, but often painfully, by forcing herself to look at her beliefs and to question them from a new, and adult perspective, she connects to a continuous thread of hope and help. One that will eventually reweave her life and her perspectives into a picture that she wouldn't have been able to see from her old ways.

When she is diagnosed and travels her journey with breast cancer, Denise comes to a place of forgiveness of self and others. She expertly draws from her life experiences and counselling education and uses a wealth of resources to explain such things as "The Biological Effects of Living in Chronic Fear", "Integrating Head and Heart", and "Balancing Feminine and Masculine Principles" to name a few. She shares her self-development with a courageousness that is open yet kind. It is this openness and honesty that encourages us to look at ourselves. Throughout life we can get sick and may develop dis-ease or illness. Our motivation to heal is often brought on by a sudden shock perpetuated by fear. Denise shows that if we are willing to love and forgive unconditionally, and if we pay attention to the whispers of intuition, our healing can also be inspired just as much by hope.

Denise develops an "Attitude of Gratitude" even for the things that didn't appear to be so wonderful at all, when she discovers a phrase that forever changes the way she looks at herself and others: "What would love do here?" Coming from the heart, a place of love, it feels safe to read, safe to think, and safe to do our own healing work, as she guides us through what often appears to feel like impossible states of awareness. We learn to unconditionally accept all of life's experiences. As she continues to discover her inner beauty, her outer beauty amplifies and she begins to become more and more aware that she indeed has the power to choose and create her own life. Because of her love and gentleness to self and others, we are encouraged to see things with fresh new eyes; like those of the unconditional love of a child.

With full awareness, Denise tells us that it is just *her* story from *her* perspective. While she retells the general information of her story, she does not get stuck in the drama of it; therefore we as the reader also do not get caught up in it; nor do we take sides. We are merely observers. Looking at the changes in her life shows us how we unconsciously make choices and how those choices connect to one another.

I am honoured and delighted to recommend *Whispers of Hope*. As you read and work through the "Tools for Transformation," wonderful thought provoking questions at the end of each chapter, they will guide you to your own discoveries if you allow yourself to process and then do what resonates with you. You are the only one who can change your world. *Whispers of Hope* will help you come back to your heart and find the peace that is always within.

Virginia Smith BGS, RT-CRA
Reiki Master Teacher/Practitioner
Canadian Reiki Association Vice-President

How to Use This Book

THE PAGES OF THIS BOOK map out the transformational journey I took from surviving to thriving! Each chapter builds on the one before, and reveals the next steps I took on my path.

At the end of each chapter you will find "Tools for Transformation". These are a series of questions designed to help you begin to transform your perception and co-create an extraordinary life. It would be helpful to set off on this adventure with a journal, to record your answers to the questions posed, as well as to document any insights you come up with along the way.

There is more than one path to peace. Within this book there are many tools that you can use. Please remember that no one else is an expert on your life. As you read the information in this book, take it in and if it moves you, touches you, or speaks to you, try it on to see if it fits for you. If it does not, set it aside. Use your gift of discernment to decide what works best for you.

You will notice I have used terms such as God, Goddess, Source, Creator, Spirit, Divine, and Universe interchangeably throughout the book. This is meant to be inclusive of the many words used to describe the loving, intelligent, conscious energy larger than our personal self – the All consciousness. Please feel free to use, or substitute, whatever word works best for you.

The only thing asked of you before you embark on this expedition of self-discovery is that you be willing to temporarily set aside any pre-conceived ideas and beliefs you may have so that you can see with new eyes.

Grab your journal, open up your heart and mind, and let's begin!

Prologue: A Fairy Tale - Life behind the Wall

The Journey from Fear to Love, Showing How We Begin to Hide Our True Selves

ONCE UPON A TIME in the Kingdom of Smoke and Mirrors there lived a king. He came from a royal family that had almost been destroyed by alcohol. One day, while on a fishing trip in the country, he met a poor young maiden in distress who captured his heart. When he returned her to her home he realised all was not well in the maiden's family. She was badly mistreated there. The king could not bear to witness the maiden's suffering and so he decided to rescue her. They were married and he carried her off to his castle on his white horse and made her his queen.

The new queen thought moving to the Kingdom of Smoke and Mirrors would be the answer to all her problems. But to her dismay, her ignorance of big city ways only served to increase the queen's feelings of low self-worth. The queen began to numb her pain with alcohol, just as her father had done.

Three years later the queen decided having children would be the magical solution to all that ailed her. Three children were born in rapid succession to the royal couple. The beautiful daughter was born first and was the apple of the king's eye. The queen knew she should love this child, but that was an impossible task for her since she did not know how to love herself. The baby was by no means the miracle the queen had counted on. Instead of solving all the queen's problems, the new princess and all her needs only compounded the queen's insecurities. This little being, who should have been welcomed into the world and loved unconditionally, bore the brunt of the queen's unhappiness.

The princess became wise beyond her years. If only she could stop crying and be quiet. Then maybe the queen would not be so angry and

3

violent all the time. 'BE QUIET' became the first row of bricks in the wall the little child began to construct around her tender heart.

But the silence left her alone in a prison of her own feelings. The princess reasoned that if only she could stop feeling lonely, stop feeling angry, stop feeling sad, stop feeling needy, stop feeling anything, the pain inside of her would end. So she did. 'STOP FEELING' became the next layer of bricks.

These two layers were not nearly high enough to shield the princess from the queen's contempt and the king's desperation at not being able to please the queen. So the child thought that if she could only be perfect maybe the king and queen would stop fighting and live happily ever after. The princess became a super achiever, the best at everything she attempted. She began to measure her own self-worth by her achievements. But the little girl was very, very careful. She attempted only that which she knew she could excel at. My God, what if she should ever fail? She would never get another chance to try to win the queen's love, and the king's adoration would surely vanish. She thought she would rather die, and so 'DO NOT EVER FAIL' became the next row of bricks.

The princess was growing into a young girl and could no longer see over the wall she was building. Despite her best efforts to be quiet, to stop feeling, and to never fail, nothing the princess did stopped the queen's abuse or lessened the king's sadness. The princess knew there must be something terribly wrong with her if her own mother did not love her.

As the queen's drinking increased she left the castle more and more often trying to find solace. The princess took on the roles of surrogate spouse to the king and surrogate mother to her two brothers. She cooked, she cleaned, she babysat, but to no avail. Instead of making the queen happy, it infuriated her and she resented the princess even more. The next row of bricks in the princess's wall became 'GROW UP—BE AN ADULT'.

The young princess was growing into a young lady and she had lost sight of who she really was. To the world outside of her walled heart she appeared to have escaped unscathed by the violence and abuse in her home. She wore her mask perfectly.

The princess became a woman of many masks and married her own masked prince. All appeared to be going well in the Kingdom of Smoke and Mirrors. Then the princess had two children of her own and the wall she had so carefully built, brick by painstaking brick, was beginning to show signs of wear. The mortar between the bricks began to crack. She found herself yelling at her children.

The princess knew if she wanted to stop the cycle of family abuse and pain she would have to start taking down the wall. But she did not know how. It had been in place for so long and kept her safe as a child. Her ego screamed that if she took down the wall she would die. But whisper by whisper, the voice of hope began to get louder...

Part I – In the Beginning

Identifying the Baggage from the Past

1. Hands

"The final forming of a person's character lies in their own hands."

Anne Frank

I DO NOT REMEMBER WHEN I STOPPED BELIEVING in fairy tales. If family photos are an indicator, then I would say sometime before my first birthday. Portraits of me at a year old are haunting. They reflect eyes that have seen more than a one year old can comprehend. Apprehension and sadness had moved in where spontaneity and joy should have resided. If there really was a happily ever after I was not able to find it at my house.

The search had been going on for as long as I could remember. Yet I really could not even define what I was searching for. There just always seemed to be an ache inside me for something different. Maybe it, whatever *it* was, would be around the next corner. Surely there had to be more to life than this. This quiet desperation, this day to day living that could not even really be called living. More like existing. What exactly was the point? It was a life defined by other people and circumstances, a life of reaction, always waiting for the other shoe to drop, a life of fear and contraction. It was lonely, devoid of true connection because I was too afraid to really open up my heart and let others in. I kept waiting for something outside of me to change so I could feel better.

My journey had been fraught with adversity including: childhood experiences of abuse and alcoholism, leaving home at 16, my father's suicide when I was 18, breast cancer at 35, and the end of a 20-year marriage when I was 42. My life path was like the twists and turns of a labyrinth, continually bringing me back to myself, giving me repeated opportunities to see the many facets of who I truly was. Really *see* them. Not just with my eyes, but with my heart and soul.

9

At this point in the journey I am finally able to answer the unspoken question, the one that has been handed down in my family for generations and was transmitted energetically with so much contempt. The question that reverberated throughout my body anytime I dared to stand in my Truth. "Who do you think you are?" I can answer that question now. I have come home to myself and I really like where I live!

It has not always been so, actually, far from it. If those who knew me as a child were to meet me now, they would find very little resemblance between the person before them and the frightened young girl I once was. I have grown from a child, feeling victimised by the circumstances of my life, to an adult who recognises I have choices, someone who has never given up hope. I have found a wellspring of love at the centre of my being and have made a conscious choice to live every day from that place. Almost all of us have grown up with less than ideal circumstances. I felt a burning desire to make sense of all that had happened in my life. I certainly do not have all the answers, but I live and love the questions. This is my story.

It all began with hands. A person's hands and how they use them will tell you more about them than an autobiography. A life path is contained in the lines of their palms. The backs will tell you their age. The texture of the skin will tell you how they labour. Is it soft and supple or hard and coarse? How well do they care for themselves? Are the fingernails well-manicured or dirty and broken? Is their touch filled with love and kindness or with fear and anger? Even though people may try to alter their appearance to give a false impression, their hands will always tell the truth. Like their fingerprints, they are totally unique. There is not another person in the world with the same blueprint for life.

If I had known to look at my parents' hands when I came into this world, I would have seen the generations of hurt and pain held in their very cells. I might have understood from my first breath their abuse had nothing to do with me. But I was a baby, dependent on those hands for my survival. The deeper understanding of their legacy of pain would elude me for years.

On the day I was born, my father's hands were soft hands; not strong hands, but steady hands and at times, almost tentative. They were kind, gentle, loving hands. They were gifted hands, brilliant hands, musical hands. They were hands that had known wealth and privilege and yet at the same time they were hands that never felt like they belonged on this earth. They felt unwanted and useless—like they were never quite good enough. They were lost hands despite their beauty and they foretold a short life.

My mother's hands told a different story in many ways, and yet the essence was very similar. Her hands were young, innocent, and afraid. They were strong and filled with rage. They spoke of hard work, poverty, and abuse. Underneath all of that there was a yearning to do it differently with her own children. It took until the end of her short life before she was able to tap into that hunger and begin to try to satisfy it. They, too, were hands that never felt good enough, and that underlying belief coloured everything they did.

My baby girl hands were a blend of the two. They were shaped like my father's and mirrored his softness, kindness, gentleness, and brilliance. They carried my mother's strength, innocence, and a desire to do it differently than the generations before her. What I inherited from both sides was the feeling of not being good enough. What hid in the shadows waiting to be claimed were the qualities of compassion, determination, the ability to see into the very heart and soul of people, and unconditional love of self and other. I spent the first part of my life gathering evidence to support the inherited mistaken belief of not being good enough. Part of my life's purpose has been to venture into the shadows, shine a light in the darkness, and reclaim the qualities that speak the Truths I forgot on the day I was born.

I finally know at the core of my being that I am okay, more than okay actually. I know there is a reason why I am here, that my life has purpose and meaning, and that I matter. There really is a happily ever after.

Tools for Transformation

- *Who do you think you are?*

- *Why not follow me on this adventure and find your Truth?*

2. Anxiety Soup

*"People who come from dysfunctional families
are not destined for a dysfunctional life."*

Bo Bennett

I HAVE BEEN TOLD I WAS A BEAUTIFUL BABY, soft, almost angelic, fair haired and fair skinned, with the most intense eyes. Eyes that saw everything, took it all in, and tried to make sense of a world that made no sense at all. My father doted on me and my mother loved and hated me in turns. Dad treated me as if I was a china doll, something precious, beautiful to behold, irreplaceable, to be handled with care. Mom, on the other hand, treated me like a rag doll, cheap, easily overlooked, dispensable, to be tossed in the corner when I was no longer useful. Neither parent looked at me as a little person with the same capacity for feeling as they had.

I was born into the end of an era where children were to be seen and not heard. This provided a sharp contrast to the very nature of being a newborn. I cried a lot and I needed a lot. The realities of caring for me were more than my mother was prepared for. She was barely more than a child herself. The more I cried and needed, the more anxious my mother became. My cries for love and belonging echoed my mother's own cries that had gone unanswered, unearthing her soul wounds and those of her mother before her. My mother told stories, and I have early sense memories, of her anxiety turning to frustration and then to anger in the blink of an eye. Luckily for me there was a woman living in the same boarding house as us, who heard my constant cries and felt moved to answer them. She would come and sit and rock me to give my mother a break. Her sure and loving touch was enough to calm me and I would stop crying. These were brief periods of respite for my mother and me, but their impact was huge. They reinforced my mother's feelings of inadequacy while simultaneously planting seeds of proof of a friendly Universe in my subconscious awareness. Those seeds would prove to be the beginning of a lifeline I clung to during some of the darkest times in my life.

I began to talk at six months of age and walk by nine months. This was a good thing, as two brothers followed my birth in rapid succession. The first when I was eleven-and-a-half months old and the second when I was two years and eight months old. My mother's feelings of self-loathing multiplied exponentially with each child. By the time her third baby was born she had abandoned any illusions that she might be a good mother and turned to alcohol to numb her pain. The role of mother quite naturally fell to me, a job I was neither qualified nor ready for.

Growing Up in a Dysfunctional Family

I lived in a world of chaos and uncertainty. My mother was like Dr. Jekyll and Mr. Hyde, and alcohol only served to intensify her extremes. There were moments when things were okay, but those moments could become dark and foreboding as quickly as storm clouds gather in the sky before a torrential downpour. Then the abuse would rain down with force and vengeance, leaving a path of destruction in its wake. I never really understood what triggered the storms, but I mistakenly suspected it was somehow my fault. I wanted so desperately to be loved and accepted by my mother. I would have done anything to try to earn that love. I did not know love was supposed to be unconditional. I began to hide those parts of myself that met with disapproval. I became an expert in studying people. I could read their faces and their bodies for clues as to their state of mind. I honed my perception and my intuition and could sense in every fibre of my being when people, places, or things were not safe.

People outside of our family commented on how well behaved and mature I was, wise beyond my years. Most never knew what went on behind closed doors. My school pictures told the story though, if anyone had taken the time to study them. They reflected a very sad and conflicted face. My eyes, my beautiful intense eyes, had become clouded and vacant. The windows to my soul were dusty and broken from neglect. I often left my body now to escape the pain. The abuse had gone beyond the physical and seeped into my mental and emotional world as well. The only way I could save the spiritual part of me was to leave. Since I was too little to physically remove myself from the source of the agony, I survived using the only option available to me; I left my body energetically until the pain stopped. A teacher once asked, "What lurks behind that smile?" Even I did not know anymore.

My childhood was a time of immense pain and fear and sadness. Even more than sad, it was heartbreaking. I guess you really could not call it a childhood at all. There was no spontaneity, or joy, or fun. I went from being a baby to an adult almost overnight once my brother was born. Instead of being nurtured myself, I was expected to take care of him. I would be sent to give my brother his bottle and my mom would find me in the corner drinking it myself. Punishment would be swift and violent. I learned it was not okay to have needs, and certainly not okay to expect to have them met. I got so used to being hit I would flinch every time my mother walked past me. She took me to the family doctor thinking the flinching indicated there was something wrong with me.

The days felt extremely long waiting for my dad to come home from work. When my father was there things were better. Just his presence lessened my fear somewhat. He never raised a hand to me. I could count on that. I adored my dad. He came home tired and frustrated from a job he hated, but he did not vent his frustration on his children. Quite the opposite, his way of dealing with his pain was to sleep. Even though he was emotionally unavailable most of the time, I put him on a pedestal. It would be many years before I began to see that even though he was not the perpetrator of the abuse, he did not do anything to stop it.

By the time my second brother came along there were no longer any child-like qualities visible in me. I had buried them deep in order to survive. Life was lonely, desperately lonely. I was an adult/child. I did not belong in the adult world and yet I was totally out of place in a child's. I felt completely on my own. I did not even know how to play, because I never had. With three children under the age of three my mom did not have time for me so I taught myself how to tie my own shoes before I started school. I taught myself to read by looking at the TV Guide and relating it to whatever show was on television at the moment. When I finally did start school I saw what an effort it was for my mother to get my brothers ready for the mile long walk there. It was stress and strain for everyone and so I decided to be brave and tell my mother I wanted to walk by myself. I thought I saw hurt and disappointment in my mother's eyes, but she agreed to let me walk on my own. I was confused. I was only trying to make my mom's life easier and yet again I thought I had upset her. It did not seem to matter how hard I tried, I could not make my mother happy. I would have given anything to make that so. I was too young to understand I had no control over another's feelings or actions. I thought if I just tried harder somehow I could make things okay. What I ended up doing was giving away my Self.

It was a childhood of not enough. Not enough time, not enough attention, not enough money, not enough food. Certainly not enough love. I came to believe I was not enough. If I were enough, surely I would have been more important to my mother than the alcohol. If I were enough my mother would not be so angry all the time and my father would not be so sad. I tried hard to make everything okay, and I thought I had failed miserably. I carried the weight of that perceived failure and the terrible secret that I was not okay wherever I was. It felt crushing. I carried it at home and became very, very quiet. I carried it to school and became a straight 'A' student. I carried it into my relationships and became a chameleon. I became whoever and whatever others wanted me to be and was the best at whatever I did. Because to be anything less would call others' attention to the secrets I was carrying. If I made a mistake and let slip what was going on at home, I was convinced they would come and take my brothers and me away. I did not even know who *they* were. But as bad as life was at home, it was familiar. We lived next door to a woman who took in foster children. She treated them like dogs. They were put in the laundry room by themselves to eat their meals. They were given beds, a roof over their heads, and meals. But they were not given human dignity. Given a choice I would rather be abused by my own mother than a stranger.

The early years of school were not any better. We lived in a one-bedroom apartment above a store. I shared a bedroom with my brothers, and my parents slept on a pull-out couch in the living room. There really was not room to have friends over, even if I had any. I was embarrassed about my mother. What if I asked a friend over after school and my mother was drunk and raging when we got home? It was bad enough to live in it, but at least I could keep the world of home and outside separate. A source of salvation for me was being able to see a world outside the chaos, live in that world whenever I could, and not mix the two; never mix the two. I did not want the rest of the world to find out where I came from and that I was not okay.

I met my best friend in grade two. She lived down the street. I loved spending time at her house. She had her own bedroom with two single beds and a television in it, and she did not have to share anything! It was decorated in beautiful soft girl colours and textures. We used to stay up in bed on Friday nights and watch Johnny Carson. When we woke up on Saturday mornings her mom would treat us like princesses. She waited on us hand and foot and made us anything we wanted for breakfast. She marvelled at how many pancakes I could eat at one sitting, not realizing I did not get homemade pancakes at home. She always said she was happy to cook for someone who enjoyed it so much. I spent lots of time there because I felt taken care of. I felt wanted there. I felt loved there. Her mom taught us how to embroider, crochet, needlepoint, and knit. She even taught us how to do yoga. We had sleepovers almost every weekend. They owned a cottage on a lake, and they often took me with them when they went there. With them I got to see a whole other world, one where I was valued for who I was.

I loved the lake and being out in nature. I felt like I belonged there. I shared my love of nature with my father. He respected the tenderness of new growth and had the patience required to nurture beauty outdoors. He grew climbing rose bushes that were the envy of the neighbours. They were his pride and joy. Perhaps they were his attempt to give what he had not experienced as a child: unconditional love and a feeling of being wanted. He loved to be on the water too. Fishing was a hobby he had shared with his own dad. It was a quiet reflective time for him. I was the only child allowed to go fishing with him because I was the one who could stay quiet in the boat and not scare the fish away. I would have done anything to spend quality time alone with my dad. From this I learned that to get the love and attention of a man I loved, I needed to be silent. When we were out fishing, my dad was so much in the moment he did not even whistle, and he loved to whistle. His whistling was not idle and pointless. It was very melodious and beautiful to listen to. I had never heard a nightingale, but I imagined it must have sounded like my dad. Oh, how I loved my dad, his kind gentle spirit, and the deep sadness he carried. I wanted so much for him to be happy. I felt that somehow I was partly responsible for his unhappiness and that it was my job to fix it. But it did not seem to matter what I tried, I could not take his sorrow away. I thought if I were a better daughter I would have known how to do that.

Our family lived a simple life by all accounts. My father worked at a low-paying job delivering prescriptions for a drug store and my mother stayed at home to raise the children. Money was tight and luxuries were nonexistent. Sometimes there was nothing in the fridge except bread, condiments, and rotting lettuce in the crisper. On those days, sustenance would come in the form of a ketchup or mustard sandwich. I hungered often, not only for food, but also for safety, love, and attention.

The inside of the apartment we called home was sparsely decorated with hand me downs. It was an odd juxtaposition of expensive cast offs from the rich customers my dad did deliveries for and bargain basement furniture that came from who knows where. One of the bargain basement chairs was covered in plastic. To protect it from what: kid wear and tear and the inevitable stains that give witness to real life being lived there; to erase any evidence of children; to disqualify their very existence; to put on airs to the world and guard against them seeing what lay beneath the surface? Maybe it was more to mask than to protect. That chair, with its plastic covering was symbolic of our family life. No one really knew exactly what lay beneath the plastic, just as no one really knew what happened in that apartment. It was made to appear shiny and new, when in fact, what lay beneath the glossed exterior was dirty and old. It was full of humiliation and rage that was to be kept out of sight at all costs. What the rest of the world did not get to see was the slow form of dying practised by the adults of the house and the mother's daily attempts to silence the voices and extinguish the light in her children. In truth, plastic did not quite cover it.

I can vividly remember every detail of the apartment: the hardwood floors throughout and the paisley patterned wool rug in the living room; the two oil paintings on the wall, with their smooth and gently-sculpted wooden frames; and the Formica dining room table with the worn chairs. Meal times around that table were evidence of poverty and reminders of *not good enough*. That energy seemed to permeate the very paint on the walls and surround and smother the life out of my family. The kitchen did not hold many good memories either. It seemed like that was where my mother was a lot of the time, at least most of the times when I needed her for something. I learned early it was a dangerous prospect to ask my mother for anything when she was busy in the kitchen. Even a request for a glass of water could result in the water being thrown in my face. It had now become dangerous to ask to have my needs met. The day when I had grown tall enough to get my own drink from the tap was a day of private celebration for me. Then I did not have to be a bother anymore.

Interestingly enough it is a challenge for me to recall smells from childhood. There are only two I can remember with any certainty. The smell of paste wax and the smell of spaghetti sauce cooking. Both were good signs; paste wax meant my mother had waxed the hardwood floors and spaghetti sauce meant my mom was cooking something she really liked. Either of these things indicated my mother was sober and in one of her happy moods for a little while. They also meant I would not get hit that day, my mom would not be angry at my dad that day, my parents would not argue that night, and my brothers would be safe. Those times did not happen very often, but when they did I knew there was a higher power out there somewhere. I was not sure where it went the rest of the time, but those infrequent times of sanity in our house were enough for me to hold on to. They helped me to navigate through the chaos, and were what I prayed for when I cried myself to sleep at night. They were the tiny whispers of hope that hinted life would be better someday, and there was something more than the insanity that was my life inside those apartment walls. I knew deep within me, without knowing the details of how, one day I would transcend the sadness and the pain and fly on my own. Somehow I would survive this.

I was very sensitive and often knew my mother's emotional storms were coming before there was even a cloud in the sky. My mother was not a full-time drunk. She was a binge drinker. I walked on eggshells all of the time so as not to do something that would trigger a binge. I did not know I was not the cause of the drinking. I just assumed it was so, as do most children of alcoholics. My mother was the nastiest when she was drunk and the abuse would alternate between physical, emotional, and verbal. Most of it landed on me. She knew me so well she knew exactly what to say to wound me to my core. She had a tongue like a knife when she was drunk, and she would often take things I shared from the deepest part of me, twist them, and stab me in the heart with them. I was very young when I put a wall up around my heart. It hurt way too much to have someone you love stomp on you whenever the mood struck them. If I could not trust my mother, who could I trust? I learned to trust no one but myself.

As I grew older my life remained centred outside of my family home. Just as I learned to leave my body to survive the abuse, I also learned to spend as little time as possible physically confined within the walls that held such sadness and fear.

My only refuge in the whole apartment was the couch in the living room. It was here I would be allowed to lay down with a blanket and watch television when I was sick. There must have been an unwritten rule about not hitting a sick child because I cannot remember ever being hit on that couch. My mother actually tried to care for me somewhat when I was sick. Consequently, I got sick a lot.

Vacations were often spent at my mother's family's farm. As much as the days were a flurry of light activities for us city kids, the nights by contrast reflected the dark. The alcohol would come out after dinner and the adults would transform. Voices would become slurred and arguments would start. Often someone ended up getting hurt. The craziness would reach its peak after the kids were sent upstairs to bed, but the flimsy construction of the old farmhouse did little to shield the younger inhabitants upstairs from what was going on downstairs. When the arguments would escalate out of control someone would head for the gun that hung on the wall near the top of the stairs. I would sit at the top of those stairs, just out of sight of the adults. I was terrified. I knew my mother was in no condition to protect herself or her children. Someone had to be the responsible adult and I got the job by default. My father stopped coming with us to the farm early on. He did not drink and he had no desire to be amongst those who did. Unfortunately, his children did not have that option until we were much older. So I would sit on the stairs and wait and pray. Pray we would all live to see the morning. When the alcohol was gone my mother would stagger up the stairs and climb into the bed she shared with me. She would hug me to her and breathe stale booze breath in my face. As much as the smells of alcoholism nauseated me, I was afraid to push her away in case she never came back. Mixed feelings coursed through me that I had neither the capacity nor the experience to deal with. I loved my mother because she was my mother and at the same time I hated her for exposing us to such danger. I would lay awake most of the night in emotional torment. I would watch for the light of morning to dawn and listen for the birds' songs. Both were signs of continuity and a stable presence that helped to ground me. When my mother finally awoke she would be hung over and impatient. There would be no talk of what happened the night before. It was as if it never happened at all. I would begin the new day with confusion and doubt in my own experience. But I continued to hope that maybe this day would be different from the one before.

Those times were crazy making. There was no one to validate my experiences. The lack of support enforced a code of silence and had me doubting my own mind. I felt alone in my struggle. It felt like the adults in my world could not be trusted, and I felt there was no one I could talk to. The combination of all of these things provided the perfect climate for sexual abuse to begin and to flourish.

My mother's uncle lived on the farm next door. He made a point of visiting when our family was there on vacation and he made a point of choosing me. I did not know he had chosen many before me, and that he would choose many after. I only knew of my own experience with him, and I felt isolated and powerless to stop it. I felt dirty and bad, sick to my stomach a lot, and I felt somehow I was responsible for what was being done to me. I steered clear of him as much as I could. When he visited, my own mother would force me to sit on his lap and give him a kiss. My mom's actions came from propriety and her need to demonstrate to her elders that she had raised an obedient child. But they only added insult to injury for me. This man took away my innocence and any semblance of childhood I might have had left. It would be years before I discovered he did the same thing to my mother when she was young, and he had also sexually abused some of my cousins. Most of them never told anyone. The ones who tried to tell were ridiculed and not listened to. The code of silence was strong and reinforced at every turn.

As I navigated the journey to becoming a young woman, I did so without a mother's guidance. I was shy, quiet, gifted academically, and I had very few social skills. I was accelerated from grade two to grade four and then attended a separate school for a grade six enrichment program. My best friend was not offered the same program and we began to drift apart. Just after I turned ten years old I walked alone to a new school where I knew no one. Feeling socially inept coming from a dysfunctional family was nothing compared to the numbing isolation I felt in the new school without my best friend. I was sad about that, and lonely.

Adding to my mistaken belief that I was walking alone in the world, my grandmother died just before I started at the new school. She was my dad's mother and I loved her very much. She spoiled me rotten and would sometimes have me over for weekends. Spending time at my grandmother's house was like living in another world. They were wealthy at one time and the house was full of beautiful things. I was allowed to play with Royal Doulton china dolls because my grandmother trusted I would take care of them. I felt special when I was with my grandmother and it was a great loss to me when she died of cancer. She lived with my family for the last months of her life. When it looked like she was nearing death my parents sent me away to my best friend's cottage for two weeks. When I came home my grandmother was dead and buried and I did not get a chance to say goodbye. After my grandmother died my family started to fall apart. She was the matriarch that kept everything pieced together.

My mom was tired of living paycheque to paycheque. This was not the dream she signed on for when she escaped the family farm at 17 years old to marry my father. She came to the big city anticipating a better life, and here they were, living in poverty. She got a part-time job working at a department store. She would often buy us gifts to make up for the neglect. Maybe she thought she could buy love. Shortly after I turned 11 my mother decided we would move into subsidised housing, where rent was geared to income. Then my parents could finally get ahead financially and eventually purchase a house of their own. My mother's dream had always been to own her own home. My parents fought about this decision constantly. Finally, my father agreed. It was on that day I saw what little light was left in my father's eyes go out for good. The decision to move would prove to be the turning point and the beginning of the descent into hell for the whole family. Changing the course of fate from then on would have been like trying to stop a roller coaster after the last car crested the peak. My father gave up all hope. I could see the resignation in his eyes and in his body language. The spark that had been dimming slowly over the years finally sputtered out. At that point he stopped fighting the *not good enough* messages he carried from before his birth. From then on he began to die a little more every day. My mother began to live the adolescence she never had. Subsidised housing opened up a whole new world and group support for her downward alcoholic spiral to rock bottom. She totally abdicated her role as a parent and her dream of owning her own home was drowned somewhere in a bottle of beer. We no longer had parents. We were out on the streets until all hours of the morning. No one seemed to notice. My mother was too busy partying with her new friends and my father was escaping his feelings of powerlessness by sleeping.

With the move I lost all my sources of outside support. I had already lost my grandmother, my father was self-absorbed in depression, and my best friend was now a three-bus trip away. Even though it was a new housing project we moved into, it was a tough neighbourhood. Life became about survival of the fittest. It was a lot like a prison environment. I learned fast and was soon able to add street smarts to my book smarts. Many kids hung out in gangs. Despite living in a townhouse development, in close proximity to many people, I continued to feel alone. I felt like I was on the outside looking in at life. I did not feel like I fit in, and truthfully, I really did not want to fit into this lifestyle. I felt like there had to be something more. I tried drinking and I tried smoking, to keep up the 'cool' image, but an altered state of being was not what I was searching for. I began to lead a double life, on the one hand trying to flow with the social norms of my environment and on the other hand going beyond the surface to unearth the deeper meaning of life. I refused to believe that what I saw around me was all there was.

I dreaded holidays and special occasions. For most people they were a cause for celebration. In our household they were valid excuses for drinking and my mother's binges lasted longer because there was more alcohol readily available. Festive dinners, if the food made it to the table at all, were not happy events. Christmas was the worst, always anticipated by us kids as a magical time, complete with our dreams for this Christmas to be different from the last. Please let this year be the one where mom is not drunk on Christmas Eve and hung over on Christmas morning. Please let this year be the one where mom is not sleeping it off after we have opened our gifts; let her be present for our enjoyment of our new toys. Please let this year be the one where we gather at the table for Christmas dinner with happiness and joy. Those were the gifts we really wanted and we never did find them in our stockings or under the tree. The saddest Christmas Eve I remember was the one where my brothers and I were sitting on the stairs watching my mom and dad argue at the front door. Mom was heading out to drink with the neighbours and dad was staying with us. He was trying to talk my mom into staying home with her kids. I will never forget the look of contempt on her face as she closed the door on her way out. We got used to disappointment and broken promises. We learned not to dream.

There were ample opportunities to stay stuck in the dysfunction. Those opportunities, coupled with parents who both abandoned their roles as caregivers, left me without boundaries and vulnerable to abuse outside of the home as well. My mother volunteered me as a babysitter to a couple who were some of her new friends. One night when the man was driving me home he insisted I sit closer to him on the front seat of the car. When we got to my house he kissed me. I was sickened and scared. I did not know what to do. These were my mom's friends and previous experience taught me my mother would believe the word of another adult before she would believe me. Feeling powerless and without support I chose not to tell anyone what happened. I just stopped babysitting for them.

I started junior high school and continued to feel like an outsider. Being smart certainly was not a ticket to acceptance, so I toned that part of myself down. I had a couple of girlfriends, but none who felt as close as my childhood friend. I spent a lot of time alone in my room listening to music. To me it was the language of my soul. The lyrics seemed to speak directly to me. This was a place where I did not feel like an outsider. Some part of me understood that if another had experienced some of what I was experiencing, then ultimately I was not alone.

I began to search for love in all the wrong places. I was 14 years old when I met my first boyfriend. Up until then I had not even so much as kissed a boy. I was more of a tomboy. Not having a mother who was available to model femininity for me, my role models were my dad and my brothers. I much preferred climbing trees and playing hockey to playing with dolls.

I could not turn to my father and brothers for advice or for guidance on what was appropriate behaviour for a girl my age. I often pretended I knew what to do because I expected I should know. I did not realise my caregivers had fallen down on their job of teaching me basic life skills. I felt like I missed a class in 'Life 101' and somehow it was my fault that I was ill-prepared to interact in the world with a healthy sense of self-esteem. Learning by trial and error was not really a great way to head into a serious relationship with a boy, but it was all I had. He was so good looking and all the girls in the townhouse complex wanted to go out with him. When he chose me, I could hardly believe my luck. It never occurred to me I was worthy of being loved. I felt like I had just won the lottery.

I needed love and acceptance and to feel like I mattered in someone's life so desperately I sold my Self in an attempt to fill those needs. He told me many things. He told me he loved me. He told me my body was beautiful. He told me he had sex with his previous girlfriend and insinuated I would somehow be *less than* if I did not agree to have sex with him. I had a lot of experience with guarding against being *less than*. I eventually allowed my need to belong to speak louder than the little intuitive voice inside of me that was saying this was not such a great idea. My angels watched out for me during that relationship. Miraculously, I never became pregnant. The whole experience was not a very romantic initiation into womanhood.

The relationship carried on for well over a year. We would get together at his house because his family was often away from home, and we had time to ourselves there. As the relationship progressed there were lots of alarm bells going off in my head. His behaviour was becoming more manipulative and controlling. We used to play-wrestle and he would often exert more force than was needed. One day he 'accidentally' hit me during one of the play fights and almost broke my nose. That was the day my intuitive voice raised from a whisper to a scream. I listened and I walked away.

Although I did not know it at the time, my life and all I was experiencing would become an opportunity to transcend the ordinary. I could choose to continue the dysfunctional hurtful patterns of the past, or I could learn what *not* to do from them and use them as stepping stones to a happier, more peaceful life.

The Biological Effects of Living in Chronic Fear

While all of these events in my life were having an impact on me physically, emotionally, mentally, and spiritually, they were also having a physiological effect inside my body I was not aware of.

From the time of my conception I was literally swimming in a neuro-chemical soup of anxiety in my mother's womb. The ingredients of this soup were the results of my mother's thoughts, beliefs, emotions, and behaviours during her pregnancy. I can only imagine what it must have been like for her to marry and come straight from the farm to a big city at 17 years of age. She had a grade eight education when she started working at a major department store for minimum wage. As time went on her dream of living happily ever after receded further and further into the distance until it eventually disappeared altogether. Her decision at 19 to have a baby was a desperate attempt to quell the anxiety that was her constant companion. With all that was going on for my mother during her pregnancy, I am certain the amniotic fluid I was swimming around in was toxic.

Dr. Paul D. MacLean, a former director of research for the National Institute of Mental Health in Bethesda, Maryland, popularised *The Triune Brain Theory*. In brief, his theory proposed an evolutionary history of the human brain. It stated that the brain consists of three layers, and each layer represents a distinctly more evolved layer formed upon the older layer developed millions of years before it. My understanding of the theory is as follows.

The first layer to develop was the *reptilian brain*. It is responsible for instinctual behaviours and the body's vital functions such as breathing, excretion, blood flow, body temperature, immune function, etc. Its job is self-preservation and it is rigid, compulsive, and active even in deep sleep. This is the part of the brain where the fight, flight, or freeze response to danger originated. A 'gut' feeling also comes from here.

The second layer to develop was the *limbic brain*. This part of the brain evolved to be more concerned with the survival of the group. It promotes bonding and connection as well as social and nurturing behaviours. It is sometimes referred to as the seat of the emotions.

The last layer to evolve was the *neo-cortex*. Its function is advanced cognition and intellectual tasks. In MacLean's theory, this part of the brain is considered the seat of reason.

At an individual level, our brain develops with us as we age. During the second trimester in utero the reptilian part of the brain is forming.

Our sense of safety and security in the world is also being formed at this stage. From birth to approximately two years of age the limbic brain is maturing. This is also the time when our foundation for self-esteem is being laid down. From approximately two to five years of age our autonomy needs begin to surface. Finally, the neo-cortex begins to develop around five to seven years of age and continues until twenty-five or so. Relationship needs become paramount from age five to approximately age eleven, and then, from age eleven to age nineteen, identity needs take centre stage.

Trauma experienced at any of these stages of brain development will significantly impact the growing child. The earlier the trauma occurs the more pronounced the effect. Trauma in utero (for example the mother's anxiety) will affect the individual's sense of personal safety. Trauma from birth to age two affects their ability to trust and connect and is internalised as 'there must be something wrong with me'. Repetitive or chronic trauma is the most damaging as it sets down neural pathways in the brain that take concentrated effort to reroute.

Generally, in our day to day lives, the three layers of our brain work together, but if circumstances become such that the brain believes we are in danger, any part can become dominant. The physically lower reptilian brain or limbic brain can hijack the higher mental functions of the neo-cortex if need be.

In his book, *When the Body Says No*, Dr. Gabor Maté talks about uncertainty, lack of information, and loss of control as being three factors that lead to stress. These were three of my constant companions while growing up in a dysfunctional family. Since the most basic reptilian part of our brain is hard wired to keep us alive, my experiences of chronic stress, triggered by emotional and physical trauma (or even just the threat of trauma), were perceived by the reptilian part of my brain as a threat, and the fight, flight, or freeze response was turned on in my body most of the time.

The fight, flight, or freeze response was not designed to be in a state of perpetual activation. It was meant to offer a short-term solution to a temporary threat. Think of the proverbial caveman about to become the sabre-toothed tiger's next meal. At the reptilian brain's signal of danger, the internal systems of the body go through some miraculous transformations. The adrenal glands flood the body with adrenalin and cortisol. Any systems not essential for life support are either slowed down or put on idle; heart and lung action accelerates, there is a constriction of blood vessels to most organs so that blood can be pumped to the muscles to get them ready to move quickly, digestion is slowed, breathing is shallow, the immune system is suppressed, there is an increase of glucose in the blood, to name a few. In normal circumstances, once the alarm is over, our bodies go through a temporary recovery phase (usually 24 to 48 hours) where we feel tired and listless as our bodily systems go back to normal functioning until the next threat. The state of hyper-vigilance required for survival in a severely dysfunctional family, where you never know when or what the next threat might be, means that the adrenal glands eventually become depleted and lose their ability to adapt to stress. This can result in constant fatigue, depression, an impaired immune system, etc.

Living in chronic fear manifested itself in my life in many ways. Experiencing my mother's anxiety when I was in the womb left me feeling unsafe all the time. The physical abuse started before I was two and contributed to my lack of trust and connection. I believed there was something wrong with me. Having the fight, flight, or freeze response triggered in my body on a consistent basis resulted in my breathing being shallow. It also took a toll on my immune system. I contracted German measles at six weeks of age and caught many childhood illnesses after that. My most persistent forms of illness were colds and tonsillitis. I would get fevers so high I would become delirious. In Louise L. Hay's brilliant book *You Can Heal Your Life*, she states that the metaphysical cause of colds is too much going on at once, mental confusion, and disorder. Tonsillitis is caused by fear, repressed emotions, and stifled creativity. I felt tired and overwhelmed all the time. Because the trauma in my family life started early and was chronic the neural pathways set down in my brain to deal with the dysfunction were deep. It has taken consistent effort for me to be able to recognise and override the reptilian brain when it kicks into action. Each time I make a conscious choice to act from a place of love rather than from that fearful place of past conditioning, I forge new neural pathways in my brain. The new pathways become the norm the more I follow them. This is an ongoing process for me.

As grim as all of this may sound, it has been my experience it is never too late to begin to turn things around. I share this information with the intent of letting you know that if you have grown up in less than ideal circumstances (which pretty much includes everyone on the planet!), then you are not alone in your experience. If you are feeling pretty crappy right now, this information might provide some insight as to how you may have arrived at this place.

Just know that wherever you are on your journey is perfect. There is a reason why this book has found its way into your hands. I honour your process and your past and I stand with you as you courageously explore ways to experience peace in your present.

Tools for Transformation

- *Make a list of the traumatic childhood experiences that you would like to turn into stepping stones to a more peaceful life. Please do not dismiss your traumas because you think they are small in comparison to someone else's. If something had a negative impact on you, it matters. Once you have completed your list, hold onto it, and we will address it in Chapter 21.*

3. It Takes a Village to Raise a Child

*"We have all known the long loneliness, and
we have found that the answer is community."*

Dorothy Day

WHEN I LOOK BACK on how my brothers and I responded to our environment growing up I am amazed at the human spirit's resiliency and capacity for love. We each handled things in our own way. It was almost as if we retreated to our own corners and lived separate lives within the same walls. When we compared stories in later years there were some things we remembered similarly, and many things only one of us could remember experiencing. We took things in and processed them through our own filters. Often we had three different accounts of the same event.

How Fear Can Turn into Anger - Either Repressed or Acted Out

What we all experienced back then, whether we knew it or not, was anger; anger at being neglected, anger at the lack of encouragement and support from our parents, anger we did not have a family life like other people, anger that the adults who were supposed to look after us were too caught up in their own pain to be present for us. Anger was a cloak we wore to cover up our fear. Fear was not something we wanted to show to the world; it would make us more vulnerable. Each of us expressed our fear differently. The brother closest to me in age acted it out. He got into trouble a lot. I remember my parents having a discussion once about sending him away to reform school. His actions

33

were a way of saying, "You're not seeing me." My youngest brother expressed his through illness. He spent many of his younger years in and out of the hospital battling asthma; his body's way of saying, "I'm suffocating here; please pay attention to me." I ate my fear and anger. From the time I was eleven and a half months old, stealing my new baby brother's bottles, food became a source of comfort for me. It was a way to satiate all my hungers. It was my way of saying, "I'm starving here." All were our desperate child-like attempts to get what we needed to survive. Needs drive behaviour and when I think about it now, we were pretty resourceful in getting our basic needs met. Sometimes it required drastic measures. Interestingly enough, each of us sought out surrogate families to belong to.

I am now able to view these experiences through new eyes. The beauty is that what separated us emotionally when we were children has become the source of what draws us together as adults. Our common experience and our love for each other bring tears to my eyes just thinking about them. We know we are there for each other now, no matter what.

The Power of Community

Eventually my father got a better-paying job and my mother ended up working full time outside the home. Finances were becoming less of an issue and so my parents decided to move out of subsidised housing and rent a two-bedroom condo. My father thought distancing my mother from her drinking friends would solve her drinking problem. It did not. She found new friends to drink with at her new job. My father's refusal to drink with her placed a wedge in their relationship early on and the distance between them continued to widen year after year. My mom also looked for love in all the wrong places and she expanded her search from new drinking partners to looking for a new romantic partner in her life. My mother was not home often and my father was sad and lonely all the time. We probably should have suspected she was having an affair, but we did not and it came as a shock when she decided to share the news with my brothers and me. I felt disgust and hatred for my mother. I wondered how she could be so selfish. I was 14 years old and thought I knew everything.

I had just entered grade ten in school when I met my new best friend in science class. She lived within walking distance of our condo. She and her family became my saving grace. They took me in as if I was one of their own and I spent most of my time there to avoid going home. I slept at home on school nights, but weekends and weekdays after school I spent with my new 'family'.

As a blended family they already had two daughters and five sons when I arrived on their doorstep. The expression, "it takes a village to raise a child" certainly applied in my case. When they opened their door and their hearts to me this family became my village. When my mother's drinking was at its worst, being cocooned in the warmth of their home saved me from a path of self-destruction that I do not even want to go down in my imagination now. They taught me there are no limits to the amount of love someone can give and that there is no upset a cup of tea will not soothe. They called me their "adopted daughter", and their willingness to be there for a young girl in trouble showed me I mattered.

Knowing That Someone Cares About You and That You Matter

My 'adopted' family was not the first to show me I mattered. The woman in the boarding house when I was a newborn took the time to soothe and nurture me. My grandmother also filled that role by loving me. My first best friend's mother spent a lot of time with me. There were several teachers in school who took the time to see me and to acknowledge some of my gifts. My elementary school principal made it possible for me to go on a field trip. We needed to be back at school early from lunch so we could leave the school for the trip. I said to him, "I can't go because there isn't enough time for me to walk home, have lunch, and get back in time." He made arrangements for me to have lunch at the home of a classmate who lived across the street from the school. He also spent time with me talking about removing the words "I can't" from my vocabulary. His lesson to me was about expanding my horizons beyond what my family taught me. Whenever the words "I can't" enter my mind now, I think of him, remember I have choice, and change my words to either "I choose to…" or "I choose not to…". My grade five and grade six teachers were sisters and they both took the time to nurture me. My grade nine English teacher commented on a paper I submitted, "…you show great promise as a student of literature." Even my youngest brother was my champion at times. When I was in grade four I was being bullied by a boy who liked me. I am not quite sure where the concept of hitting a girl to show her you like her came from, but this boy had mastered it. It got to the point where I did not want to go to school anymore. My brother was in kindergarten at the time. We were outside at recess and the boy was bullying me again. My brother, who probably weighed all of about twenty pounds soaking wet, came flying across the school yard and jumped on the boy's back. He started pounding on him telling him, "Leave my sister alone!"

Sometimes the smallest gesture by someone was enough to help me remember the truth of who I was: a kind word, a smile, taking the time to acknowledge my presence. These were the things that touched my heart and made a difference in my life. They may not have been big in the world's eyes, but they were huge in mine. These people got to be earth angels and weave strands in the invisible net of support that carried me through my early years.

Differentiating from Our Families of Origin

I spent most of my adolescent and young adult years living in reaction, either trying not to be like my mother or else subconsciously repeating her behaviour. While living this way I did not get to know my true self, live in the moment, or find out what I stood for.

My way of managing the anxiety created by dealing with my family was to cut myself off from them. I could do that physically, emotionally, mentally, and spiritually. Physically, I stopped going to the family farm when I was around 12 or 13. That way I did not have to be part of what went on there. I left home to live in my own apartment at 16 years of age. Having my own space, free of the effects of alcohol, was my dream for as long as I could remember. When I got my first full-time job, I made that dream a reality.

Emotionally, I could cut myself off from people standing right in front of me. If the anxiety of our encounter overwhelmed me, I would vacate the space energetically. My mother-in-law said it best when she commented that there would be a point in our conversation when she knew the wall was up and she could no longer reach me. It was like the lights were on, but nobody was home.

My mental vacations from what was happening in the moment were many. I stayed in my head analyzing things to death in order to distance myself from feeling what was going on in my heart. I used thinking and doing as ways to avoid being.

Spiritually, I cut off from Source often. For the first part of my life I was not consciously aware there was a Source. As I got older I developed a skewed concept of God. We were not a religious family, and my idea of God was an old man with a white beard sitting on his throne in the clouds somewhere. God was a he, and He was a punishing God that used fear to keep people in line. I was angry with God. If there was a God, how could He have let those things happen to us? I refused to have that kind of God be part of my life.

All of these ways of trying to avoid feeling the anxiety that was my constant companion were actually keeping me stuck in the past. I began to learn that differentiating from my family of origin did not mean cutting off from them and trying to leave them behind. It meant learning how to be in emotional contact with them while simultaneously remaining autonomous in my own emotional functioning. It meant learning how to respond to situations while openly accepting my own emotions and not becoming what someone else needed me to be in order to lower their anxiety or mine.

Tools for Transformation

- *How do you manage anger? Do you act it out, keep it in, or ride it out. The next time you experience anger see if you can dig a little deeper to find out what emotion is beneath the anger?*

- *Who was part of your village growing up? How can you create a supportive network of people around you now?*

- *Was there someone in your past who believed in you? How did you feel when you were with them? What small step could you take today to show the child within you that you believe in yourself?*

- *Is the language you use every day limiting your experience? Notice the number of times you use words like: can't, should, I have to. Can you take ownership of your experience and change what you say to indicate you have choice in every moment?*

- *What are your coping strategies to alleviate anxiety? When anxiety is present in your body, see if you can take some time to sit with it and see what its message is for you. How long can you sit with it before you think you have to 'do' something with it? Observe how this differs when you are alone with the anxiety and when you are in relationship with someone and there is anxiety between you.*

4. Could I Have Saved My Father?

"To her the name of father was another name for love."

Fanny Fern

IT GOT TO THE POINT where my mother was seriously considering leaving my father and moving into her own apartment. I do not know if my mother and father talked about this or if my father knew intuitively something was wrong. In any case, he began to sleep much more. It became harder each day for my mother to wake him up in the mornings to get him to go to work. My dad thought the sun rose and set on my mom and, for him, a life without her was a life not worth living. The day came when he would not get out of bed at all. My mother called an ambulance and I watched, frozen in the background, as the paramedics loaded my father onto a stretcher and took him away. I could not make him better and I could not stop what was happening.

He was committed to a psychiatric hospital and he was there for a long time. I did not go to visit my dad often; seeing him in that place tore at the fabric of my soul. It was not my father I saw there; it was a grotesque shell of the man I knew. The sadness and despair of the hospital engulfed me and I could not get through to my dad. His body was there, but the essence of who he was, was somewhere else. We went to the hospital as a family for counselling sessions but my father's mental health did not improve. The doctors decided to give him electric shock therapy. I found out this was not his first nervous breakdown. He was hospitalised once before in his late 20s just after he met my mother. He received shock treatments then too. No one ever talked about that in my family.

Eventually my mother did the only thing she knew how to do. She told my father she still loved him and she would not leave him. After that, my dad slowly began to get better, and within a few months he came home armed with anti-depressants. He was painfully thin and almost beyond recognition. Our family dog did not even know him at first. When he walked in the front door the dog sniffed his unfamiliar hospital scent. But when he spoke, she knew the sound of his voice and nearly turned herself inside out with ecstasy at having him back home.

Life slowly began to return to the way it had been before. My mother was continuing her search for happiness outside of herself and decided we needed a change of environment. She wanted to move to an apartment with three bedrooms so my parents, my brothers, and I each had a bedroom. The only catch was the new apartment building did not allow pets. The family dog was getting old. My dad was given the job of taking her to be euthanised, as my mother did not drive. It was a sad day for the family and especially for my father. He had such a soft spot in his heart for animals.

It was not long after we moved into the new apartment that my mother changed her mind about staying with my dad. She was going to move out after all. My brothers and I chose to stay with my father. We watched the months tick by as our dad valiantly tried to make a life for himself without his wife. He even tried going out on a date once, but his heart was not in it.

After a while I made a choice to go ahead with my plan to move out on my own. The idea of moving started out to be mostly about getting away from my alcoholic mother. Even though my mother was gone, I had prepared energetically for this move for so long it took on a momentum of its own and I followed through with it. The brother closest in age to me spent a lot of time hanging out with his friends away from home. My youngest brother was the only one who remained at home consistently with my dad.

I visited my father as often as I was able. Between my full-time job and spending time with the man who was now my fiancé, those visits were not frequent. It was hard to witness the sorrow that was so much a part of my dad now. I could sense he was heading into that downward spiral of darkness and depression again, to that private place of anguish where no one could reach him. I felt powerless, but I also knew I had to do something to try and bring him out of it. Another of my mother's dreams was that the family would someday go to Miami for a vacation. That dream had not come true. Since I was working a full-time job I decided to save some money. I promised my dad I would take him to Disneyworld for Father's Day in June, a gift to him to show him how much I appreciated everything he had done for me all my life. I wrote my surprise invitation in his birthday card in April. In May, on a weekend when he knew there was not a chance he would be found in time, he overdosed on his anti-depressants and took his own life. He was 52 years old.

Life changed forever for me on the day I received the call that brought the news of my father's death. When I hung up the phone a primal scream of anguish began to rise up from deep inside of me. It made it as far as my throat before I choked it back. I was afraid if I let it out I would never stop screaming. I was 18 and I felt as if my heart had been wrenched from my chest. It hurt to breathe, it hurt to move, and it hurt to be alive when the man I loved the most in the world was gone. My brothers and I went with my mother to claim my father's body at the morgue. Other than his clothes, the only thing he had on him at the time of his death was his wallet. They handed that over to us. In it were his driver's licence and a picture of me.

My brothers and I planned his funeral in a state of shock. It was a time of disbelief and everyone was looking for someone to blame. There was no suicide note. Anyone who loved my dad wanted some explanation. Most passed judgement on my mother and declared her guilty. The consensus was if she had not left him, he would still be alive. I silently joined the ranks of the accusers. Even some of the people my father worked with were nasty to my mom during visitation at the funeral home. When it was all over, my brothers and I stood together at my dad's graveside as we had never stood together before. I think we realised we were all we had left. On that day, along with our father, we buried our dreams of a happy family. I never told my mom how I felt.

My Move to the Land of 'If Only'

I experienced my own breakdown of sorts after my dad's funeral. I could not find any meaning in life and thought a change of scenery and a new start would soothe the ache inside of me; my mother had been a good role model on seeking peace externally. I quit my secure, well-paying job, left my fiancé, and moved to Calgary, Alberta to live with my cousin and her girlfriend. I was a lost soul, wandering through life, but not in it. Once again, I was trying to make sense of something that made no sense at all. I felt like there must have been something I could have done to prevent my father from committing suicide. I spent a lot of my time and energy in the land of 'if only'; if only I had visited him more often; if only I had come to visit him that weekend; if only I had not moved out on my own and stayed at home with him; if only I had been a better daughter. Staying in 'if only' kept me in my head and out of my heart, the place where I felt the pain would swallow me alive.

The move to Alberta turned out to be for only six months, but it was eye opening nonetheless. I found that rather than leaving my pain behind me, I carried it with me wherever I went. I continued to feel intense sadness for the loss of my father's kind, gentle presence in my day-to-day life. I mourned for a future we would not have together: him walking me down the aisle at my wedding, him being a grandfather to my children, and me knowing there would always be one man who loved me unconditionally.

One of my father's favourite pop songs was Kansas' *Dust in the Wind*. The lyrics, "All we are is dust in the wind." always reminded me of him. The apartment I lived in looked out at the Rocky Mountains in the distance. Nature served to ground me. Compared to those beautiful, solid, timeless structures, my problems were really a speck in the grand scheme of things. Dust in the wind, so to speak.

The time away helped me to begin to settle into a life without my father. Then the day came when I longed for home. I was still spending a lot of time in the land of 'if only,' no matter where I was geographically. It was just as easy to do that in familiar surroundings, so I moved back to Ontario. As the months passed, it became a little easier to breathe, to move, and to be alive without my dad. The loss of my father reminded me to live each day to the fullest.

My breakdown had, in essence, become a breakthrough of sorts. I was moving on to another phase of my life. When I was a young girl my dad wrote his version of a Stephen Grellet quote in my autograph book, "I shall pass this way but once. Any kindness, therefore, that I can do for any human being, let me do it now. Let me not defer it or neglect it for I shall not pass this way again." In the aftermath of his death I really understood this saying. He had shown me life could be short and we do not always get a second chance to show someone we care. It became my new mantra.

It took me twenty years, and the suicide of a good friend's grandson, before I finally began to understand that on that long-ago day in May, my father made a decision that had nothing to do with me. There was nothing I could have done to stop it. His suicide did not mean he did not love me or I was not a good enough daughter. It meant he was tired of living and it was time for his spirit to go on to the next part of its journey.

Tools for Transformation

- *Do you have some 'if onlys' weighing you down? Make a list of all you can think of. Now I would like you to make a ceremony of burning the list. Take it outdoors and use a burning pot of some sort so that you can keep the fire and the ashes contained. As it is burning, imagine releasing the energy attached to each 'if only'. This will begin to free the energy you have invested in the past and make that energy available for use in your present. You can do this on your own or invite a friend or a group to take part in the exercise with you.*

- *Are there times in your life when you feel like you have had a breakdown? What resources did you use to carry on? Is it possible to change your perception about those times and reframe them from breakdowns to breakthroughs? How did what happened alter your views and/or the course of your life in a positive way?*

- *Have you ever attempted a geographical cure? Did relocating permanently resolve whatever was ailing you?*

5. I Married My Mother!

"The events of childhood do not pass, but repeat themselves like seasons of the year."

Eleanor Farjeon

WHEN I RETURNED FROM CALGARY the relationship between my mother and I continued, on the surface, as if nothing had happened. The time and distance served to put a tentative Band-aid over my wound of losing my dad and believing my mom was to blame. I had learned not to trust my mom with things that were near and dear to my heart. Consequently, we never did talk about what happened with my dad. I thought forgiving or forgetting was impossible. I did my best to swallow my hurt and get on with my life.

I was hired back at the company where I worked before my move. I got into a relationship fairly quickly that only lasted a couple of years. I was sitting at home alone shortly after the breakup, feeling sorry for myself, when a friend from work called to invite me to a party she was having. I wanted to stay home, but I allowed her to talk me into going. There were a lot of people I knew from work there, and also some people I had not met before. A few of the men had recently returned from a contract job in Saudi Arabia. I was attracted to one of them and we began dating. He was divorced, financially independent, and was living in his own townhouse. I always said I would not date anyone I worked with because the office politics got too complicated. As it turned out, we did work in the same office, even though I had not seen him there before. Soon after, the company transferred him to a different city, which made things easier at work but more complicated on the dating front.

We were managing the weekend commute back and forth to see each other fairly well. Then one day he called me at work and said he was thinking about signing up for a two-year contract back in Saudi Arabia, and asked if I would consider going with him. He said he would give me time to think about it, as it meant leaving my friends, my family, and my career behind in Canada for two years. I did not need to think about it. I was head over heels in love with this man and distancing was something I was good at. After I hung up the phone, I thought about the fact that Saudi religious law would not allow us to live common law there. I called him back and asked him if going to Saudi together meant we would be getting married. He said that was the case, but he had planned on proposing in person rather than over the phone!

I could hardly believe all of this was happening to me. I was going to marry the man I loved, lack of money would no longer be a concern in my life, and we would be travelling thousands of miles away to live in another culture. I was excited! I was not even aware I was recreating and beginning to live my mother's dreams.

Everything happened fairly quickly from that point on. We were supposed to be ready to leave for Saudi by the beginning of September and it was now mid-August. We had a couple of weeks to collect the loose ends of our lives, plan a wedding, and get married. Luckily our departure date was extended to mid-September. Amazingly enough everything came together. I found a dress I loved, off the rack, and it fit perfectly. My new fiancé's friend was an amateur photographer who did our pictures for us as a wedding gift. We were even able to arrange flowers at the last minute. It felt like this union was meant to be. It was a small wedding performed by a minister in the chapel at city hall. There was room for 20 people and so we said our vows surrounded by immediate family and a few very close friends. My father, from my 'adopted' family, was the one to give me away at the ceremony. Afterwards, we went as a group for a beautiful dinner at a restaurant on the outskirts of the city. It was an intimate gathering and it was perfect. We arrived at the restaurant at dusk. This is my favourite time of day. A little more than a month after my 23rd birthday we became husband and wife. There were some lovely pictures taken of us just as the sun was going down.

I Thought We Were Supposed to Live Happily Ever After

Trouble began long before we said, "I do," but in increments so small I did not notice them as they occurred.

I looked into his beautiful blue eyes on the night we met and I could see into his soul. I sensed he was a good man and yet there was an air of mystery and distance surrounding him. That was the part that drew me to him. I thought I could lessen the distance if I loved him enough; that I would be able to reach him behind his wall. Probably in some way I was trying to make up for not being able to save my dad. In hindsight it really was not love I was offering at all. It was actually arrogance and naiveté on my part; arrogance in presuming he was broken and I was the one who could fix him, and naiveté around the purpose of relationship. In those days I subconsciously looked at marriage as two incomplete people coming together to find what they lacked in each other. Today I look at intimate relationship with a significant other as a spiritual partnership. In his book *The Seat of the Soul*, Gary Zukav defines the spiritual partnership archetype as a "partnership between equals for the purpose of spiritual growth". Spiritual growth was not what we were up to in our marriage. We were not two whole people coming together to support each other in our growth. We were more about stagnation and keeping the status quo; maintaining emotional distance worked for both of us back then.

My mother-in-law, who lived out of town, came for a visit shortly before the wedding. While she and I were sitting and talking, she casually mentioned she had never heard her son say he loved me. Not exactly something a bride-to-be wants to hear just before the big day! But I did not ask him about it. I was too busy making sure I did not have a relationship like my parents had. I did not want conflict. In my mind conflict meant the beginning of the end of a relationship. I did not ask him about a lot of things. I entered the marriage with my eyes wide shut. My childhood prepared me well. I was a chameleon; I would be whatever he wanted and needed me to be. There would be no rocking of the boat in this marriage. I had fallen into my childhood trap of believing that if I could make him happy then I would be happy.

Alcohol was always present. Since we mostly saw each other on weekends there would sometimes be a drink in the afternoon, or the drink with dinner, and/or maybe the drink(s) after dinner. It did not look like the binge drinking alcoholism I experienced with my mother, so I really did not see it as a problem. But deep down inside it was a problem for me. Regardless of the form it took, even one drink every day was enough to keep us from being completely emotionally available for each other. On more than one level I was marrying my mother. My husband-to-be helped me to maintain emotional distance. I was seeking something outside of me to make me happy, and a part of me believed I could make this relationship have a happier ending than the one with my mother. If I loved him enough surely he would make me more important than the alcohol.

Tools for Transformation

- *Do aspects of your current or past relationships mirror the relationship you had with either of your parents?*

- *Have any of these patterns of relating gone on in previous generations in your family?*

6. Geographical Cure (the Sequel)

"There's no place like home. There's no place like home.
There's no place like home."

Dorothy in the movie *The Wizard of Oz*

WE EXPERIENCED SOME PROBLEMS getting our entry visas for Saudi and we did not leave Canada until November 2nd. This did not cause either of us to have any doubts. We were convinced we were doing the right thing at this point in our lives. What an incredible opportunity. The plan was that we would be travelling extensively while we were away; we would have the first two years of our married life to get to know each other without in-law interference, and by the time we returned to Canada we would have saved enough money to pay cash for a house. With these ideas in my mind we departed for our new life. We stopped for a few days in London, England on the way over and then flew to Jeddah, our point of entry into Saudi. I went to a two-day orientation session set up by the company to ease my transition into this new culture. As much as they tried to prepare me for some of the realities of living in Saudi, I still had romantic *Lawrence of Arabia* notions tucked away in the back of my mind!

Life in the Kingdom of Saudi Arabia

I remember the night we arrived in the Kingdom as if it were yesterday. The airport scene in Jeddah was like nothing I had ever seen, heard, or smelled before. Hundreds of men of every nationality and dress you could imagine were all jostling for position at one of the three wickets trying to sort out their tickets for the next leg of their journey. Almost everyone was speaking Arabic, a language I was unfamiliar with. The potpourri of expensive cologne, unwashed bodies, and dirt was an assault to my senses. My biggest shock was the Saudi women who were standing out of the way of the mayhem with their children. I was told they would be covered in black. I thought that meant I would be able to see their faces, or at least their eyes. But they were completely cloaked from head to toe. The only things exposed were their hands and their shoes. I later learned that this mode of dress was called a burqa. It consisted of a loose enveloping black outer cloak-type garment called a jilbab worn over their usual daily clothing. Added to this was the head covering (hijab) and the face veil (niqab). The burqa encapsulated modesty, privacy, and morality. I do not know how they could see to walk. I was not prepared for the sameness, the shapelessness, and the total loss of identity. It was such a contrast to how Western women use external attributes to define themselves. Yet I was told by some of the women there that they appreciated the anonymity. It was a source of safety for them.

I knew my mode of dress would need to conform to their religious laws and customs. It would be floor-length skirts and dresses, long sleeves, and no ankles or wrists showing. All of this was covered by an abayah (a loose robe-like black cloak that covered everything but head, hands, and feet). I was also advised to cover my hair. But my one form of rebellion to being assimilated was to not cover my head.

We finally got on our domestic flight to Riyadh late that night. When we arrived in Riyadh airport I realised Jeddah was much more liberal. After the baggage was off loaded from the plane, we discovered one of our bags was not there. I stood in the middle of the grungy airport with our other bags while my husband went to try to locate our missing suitcase. It was late at night and I was the only woman there. I had never felt so conspicuous in my life. All eyes were on me. Now I thought I knew what a sacrificial lamb might feel like before the slaughter. The suitcase was in the lost baggage room and finally we proceeded to customs. The ritual we went through there has been unmatched in any other country I have travelled to. They searched every suitcase, top to bottom, checking for alcohol, contraband food, books or magazines with pictures of scantily clad women, and anything else that could be construed to be against the laws of Islam. These things would be confiscated if found.

Once we cleared customs we headed off to the walled compound that would be our new home. It was too dark to see much. The next morning another couple, who also lived in the compound, came and picked us up to go grocery shopping. It certainly was jarring to see Riyadh in the light of day. The landscape was devoid of colour. It consisted of piles of dirt, sand-coloured villas, and construction sites as far as the eye could see. Everywhere there was evidence of a country in transition. They were an oil-rich country whose quick fortune had seemingly catapulted them from the 14th century on their Hegira calendar, to the 20th century on our Gregorian one. They had the money to pay for the best. We saw recently built, beautiful, modern architecture next to piles of rubble that had not yet been developed. There was a large transient population of workers hired from third world countries to do the labour. The traffic was like nothing I had ever seen before. Many nationalities driving together, each following (or not following) their own pre-conceived rules of the road. It was total insanity. Cars went through stop signs and red lights. Left turns were made from the right lane and vice versa, and the horn honking was incessant. Amazingly enough we made it to the grocery store unscathed. We learned to do our shopping in between the prayer calls, which happened five times a day. The whole country stopped to pray at those times and businesses would shut down to observe prayer times.

The compound we lived in was like a small walled city, built specifically for the employees and families of the company my husband worked for. The men went off to work Saturday through Thursday and then had Fridays off. Women were not allowed to work there legally unless they entered the country on a work visa as a nurse or a teacher. All of the women in our compound accompanied their husbands to

Saudi and did not have a work visa. We entertained ourselves as best we could during the day. There was much to do within the walls. There were two Olympic-sized pools (one for adults and one for families), squash and tennis courts, and a clubhouse where many types of classes were organised by the residents. There were also buses that would take us to the downtown souks (open air market places) each weekday morning.

Despite all the available activities time seemed to pass slowly. I think I was one of the youngest wives on the compound. Shopping was not really my thing and the pools were often empty because the scorching temperatures were not conducive to being outdoors for any extended length of time. I did lots of crafts and eventually forced myself beyond my introverted nature to get out and meet people.

There were no movie theatres, restaurants, or cultural activities in the country so weekend entertainment consisted of rotating dinner parties with friends in the compound. Despite being told there was no alcohol in the Kingdom, all the ingredients were available to make your own. Of course wherever things are banned there will always be enterprising people who find ways to create a black market for them. The problem was we never really knew the quality of the product we were getting. Often the alcohol ended up to be a much higher proof than we were used to. There seemed to be something in human nature that made us want something more when we were told we could not have it.

The company was very good about making sure we left the country every four months for rest and relaxation; twice for short trips (seven to ten days) and once for an annual trip back to Canada (two to three weeks). The trips were really necessary. The Saudi culture was vastly different from our own in so many ways that getting away from it periodically helped fortify people to finish out their contracts.

We travelled to some amazing locations we would not have had the opportunity to do otherwise. Our trips included many places in the Far East, Africa, and Europe. We even brought my brothers over to Zurich to join us for a driving tour of Switzerland, Austria, and Germany. That was one of my favourite trips. It was so good to be able to see them. I really missed them while we were gone. My next favourite was the Christmas my husband and I spent in a picturesque village in Switzerland called Grindelwald. On Christmas Eve we walked up the little hill in the town to the church for the Christmas Eve service. It was a beautiful moonlit night with huge snowflakes softly falling. The kind of cold, crisp night where you can hear your footfalls crunching in the snow. I even remember the outfit I wore. I still have it hanging in my closet more than 25 years later. It helps me to remember the happier times in our marriage. Some things are hard to let go of! As for the rest of the trips, I look forward to visiting those places again. I am sure I would appreciate them more now than I did in my early 20s. As enticing as some of the places were, the truth was I really did not care where we travelled as long as we got out of Saudi's restrictive environment for a while. Consequently, I did not fully appreciate the amazing opportunity I was handed at the time.

Following the rules in a fundamentalist Muslim country involved many things most of us had no prior experience with. Any information we received within the Kingdom was censored. Their reason for doing this was to preserve their culture and protect their citizens from what was deemed an immoral Western influence. The local newspaper only carried local stories with a definite fundamentalist slant. The few Western magazines available in the country had all of the female body blacked out with a marker. All you would be able to see were their faces. Because women were not allowed to work, all of the clerks in stores were male. Grocery shopping was interesting too. Most of the products in the store had to be shipped into the country and supply did not always meet demand. An item would be available one day and then you would not see it again for months. We learned to stockpile grocery items we liked when we found them. It took a while to get over that once we got home to Canada. People looked at me strangely when I would put six of something in my shopping cart. I had forgotten I was back home and the product would most surely be available next time I went shopping!

Crime was not tolerated. There was a place in downtown Riyadh where justice was served. Expatriates nicknamed it "chop-chop square". Sentences for crimes were carried out publicly. The Saudi legal system used capital and corporal punishment. This could include amputation of hands or feet, or public floggings. Women could be stoned to death for adultery. Punishment could also be delivered outside the official justice system for things like murder or accidental death. Retribution could be sought by the victim's family either in an eye for an eye format or through blood money (money paid to the victim's family by the family of the accused). Traffic accidents were settled on the spot by the police. Damages were assessed, blame was portioned out, and if you were at fault you had to pay then and there or be hauled off to jail. Consequently most Western men always travelled with a substantial amount of cash.

Most of my husband's challenges there were work related. The Canadians from our company were brought over on a work training contract. They were the experts in their field and the Saudis sought outside expertise in many areas to bring their country up to par with the rest of the modern world. In most large companies you would find a Western manager working with a Saudi counterpart. The Western manager had been hired for a contract term to train his Saudi counterpart to do the job. The challenge with this arrangement was that the Saudi man usually had a much different value system and work ethic than the Western manager. We were trained work comes first and, if there is any time left over, then you can spend time with your friends and/or family. For Saudis it was the exact opposite. Their family and social life came first and work was fit in around that. As you can imagine, this caused great stress for the Westerners who felt like they were failing at the job they were hired to do. At the end of our two-year contract, my husband was offered an eight-month extension to complete the training. We discussed it in depth. In the end money won out and we decided to stay the extra eight months. It was eight months too long for me. My husband, on the other hand, would have

54

stayed longer. There was something about the country that called to him.

Learning That Money Does Not Buy Happiness

At first I enjoyed my time not working. I had a full-time job pretty much from the time I was 16 and having time off was a welcome rest. Shortly after we arrived in the Kingdom I found out some women were working illegally off the compound. They were taking quite a risk because, if they were caught, they and their husbands could be sent home. After we were there for five months I decided to go to work too. We had just come back from Thailand; our first trip out of the country. Leaving the confines of Saudi for the gentle exotic beauty of Thailand was wonderful, but coming back was a different story. I sank into a melancholy. I felt worse than I did before we left and thought I needed a change of pace. Since money was one of the main reasons we came to Saudi, I reasoned that the extra money I would earn would help. In addition to that I was not adjusting well to my loss of independence and personal income. I was considered my husband's property there, and that did not sit well with me. Women were not allowed to drive or be in the company of a man who was not their husband. Consequently, we became almost totally dependent on our husbands. Bit by bit I was losing confidence in myself and I wanted to do something to get it back.

Working did not turn out exactly as I planned. Rather than being a ticket to independence it became an exercise in frustration and a test of my integrity. While my husband experienced frustration around his co-worker's level of commitment to work, I had the exact opposite experience. The office I worked in as an administrative assistant had a Saudi man who was totally committed to his job and his highly-paid, contracted Western counterpart was hardly ever there. When he was there a lot of the business he conducted was personal and not for the company. I did my best to stick it out, and I lasted about a year. It got to the point where I could no longer work for the Western counterpart and I asked for a transfer to another department. After six months in the new job I put in my resignation. It was a decision I wrestled with for quite a while. Could I be bought? Exactly how much of myself was I willing to sell for the almighty dollar (or Saudi Riyal, as was the case here)? I finally realised I was getting up every morning and dreading going to work. My body, mind, and spirit were not at ease. As much as I thought earning the extra money would make me happy, I realised working in an environment where I was going against my values and beliefs every day was actually making me sick.

Living in a culture so vastly different from my own taught me a lot. I certainly learned to appreciate the freedom we have as women in the Western world. I also learned a lot about tolerance and nonjudgement. Even though the Saudi way of life was vastly different from what I was used to, that did not make it wrong. They were a generous and loyal people. Their idea of putting family and fun before work is a much more soul satisfying way to live life than the way we drive ourselves to perfection in the pursuit of external sources of happiness. I think if we chose to put family first and work second it would go a long way toward bringing peace to our planet. I sometimes wish I could go back for a visit for a few weeks. I would love to see how, and if, things have changed. I wonder if they were able to maintain their family oriented way of life or whether the pressure to become part of a Westernised world destroyed that part of their culture. It would be lovely to meet up again with some of the Saudi friends I made there. I did make some life-long friends with other couples living in our compound as well. We began by bonding over our unique, common experience and then developed close relationships that remain to this day.

Tools for Transformation

- *What is your experience of home? Is it a place and/or is it inside of you?*

- *Has the pursuit of money been a motivator in any of your decisions? If so, how did those decisions pan out? Did money deliver on its promises?*

- *Are there areas of your life where you might be selling part of your Self in exchange for money?*

7. My Mom's Breast Cancer Diagnosis

"We are not held back by the love we didn't receive in the past,
but by the love we're not extending in the present."

Marianne Williamson

THROUGHOUT OUR TIME IN SAUDI I sent letters to my mother every now and again. They were filled with descriptive details of our day-to-day life, but there were no words wasted on emotions or personal sentiments. I guess you could call them duty letters. The dutiful daughter writing to her mother. Our conversations were always about surface things, not about anything that really mattered. Writing the letters reminded me of all the years I stood forlornly in the card aisles of stores looking for a card for her birthday or for Mother's Day. Hallmark did not seem to have any greeting cards that said, "I hate you for making my childhood a living hell, and have a happy birthday." It was always a dance between saying what I really wanted to say and not wanting to insult her. My heart ached for the kind of mother they were describing in those cards. After I read each one and dismissed those that were sappy, or love and praise filled, I would settle on a generic card that wished her the best. My integrity would not allow me to lie by sending a card that acknowledged her for loving things she had not done.

The day came when our contract in Saudi was finished and we began preparations for our final trip home. We decided to stop off in Egypt on the way and then spend some time in the United Kingdom visiting with friends in England before carrying on to Scotland. In the hotel in Egypt I tossed my abayah in the garbage and said goodbye to the oppression of Saudi. I was preparing to reacquaint myself with the freedom of going home. While browsing in a small tartan shop, along a cobblestone walkway, just outside of Edinburgh Castle, I discovered

Cunningham was a name of Scottish descent. I always assumed it was English. When I told my mom about it after we got home she said she thought the Cunningham clan originated in Scotland and were driven out of Scotland into England. I was surprised by how little I actually knew about my own family history. In that shop I caught a glimpse of being connected to part of something much bigger than my little family back in Canada. I found a part of my lineage on another continent I knew nothing about. It helped me to begin to broaden my context of who I actually was and where I came from.

We found out before we left Saudi that we would not be posted back to the same city we lived in prior to our contract. Our new home town would be a four-hour drive away from my mom, which suited me just fine. She had married the man she was living with at the time of my dad's suicide. It was not a match made in heaven, but my mother finally got her dream of living in a house. My stepfather made the mistake of trying to play dad to my brothers and instil the discipline in them he thought my father neglected. Needless to say that did not go over well. My brothers and I tolerated him to try and keep peace in the family, but he was not respected by any of us. A few continents away was the ideal amount of space but a four-hour drive would now have to do.

I found the return from Saudi much more difficult than going there had been. On the trip there I was expecting life to be much different from my life in Canada. I was not expecting to have a challenge coming home. I can only liken it to having been in a prison environment for two years and eight months and then being released and trying to reintegrate back into society. Everyone we knew had carried on in their lives without us. Things had changed, people had changed, and we had been in a holding pattern. We needed to tell our stories in order to begin to assimilate our experience, but we had just lived something most people could not relate to. Our stories fell on deaf ears after a while and we found the only people we could reminisce with were those who had been in Saudi too. It seemed that coming home was easier for my husband than it was for me. He was the one working at a job loosely based on what he had been doing at home. I entered Saudi as an independent woman and that independence was stripped away a little at a time. When I got home I was afraid to drive because I had not driven the whole time we were away. For nearly three years I had not paid a bill or been responsible for my own finances. I had been living a sheltered life. My self-confidence was at an all-time low. I was on a leave of absence from work while we were in Saudi and the company found me a job three weeks after we came home. I went back to work but was not even sure of myself there anymore. At one point I wanted to take a business administration course at night school. I almost allowed my fear of driving to stop me. In the end I forced myself to get out of the house and go. Things did improve with time, but I remember thinking the company could have put on a re-entry orientation session too.

Our lives were going well. The four-bedroom house we built cost a little more than we had in savings so my income was coming in handy. Eventually I got promoted to management and the day came a couple of years later when we paid off our small mortgage. We were living on easy street. Our jobs paid well, we owned a new house that was fully paid for, and we were both driving new cars. Then the baby discussions began. We were in a financial position where I could stay home with the baby if I chose to, and that was important to me. We went back and forth on this issue in Saudi. First I was ready and he was not. Then he was ready and I was not. Now we finally agreed it was time to start trying. We thought it would probably take quite a while to get pregnant as I had been using oral contraceptives for many years. Imagine our surprise when just a few months after going off the pill I discovered I was pregnant! I was 29 years old.

I loved being pregnant. The initial three months of nausea were not great but once they subsided I felt amazing. The first flutter of life in my womb was a magical experience. Each day I marvelled at the being growing in my ever expanding stomach. My baby belly seemed to be all out in front of me, which people told me was an indicator I was carrying a boy. That, plus the doctor's conversations about the slower speed of my baby's heartbeat, had me pretty much convinced I was going to have a son. I was okay with that. Since I had grown up a tomboy I really did not know what to do with a girl. I worked until a month before my due date and then took the last month off to get ready for the new addition to our family. We decorated the nursery in neutral colours: soft beiges, greens, and yellows. We filled it with love. Stuffed animals and all of the wonderful gifts we received from friends and family lined the shelves and the floor. Then we anxiously awaited the birth of our first child.

I Am Still too Angry to Forgive

During my pregnancy my mother and I rarely exchanged phone calls. We had never really done that over the years. There were the obligatory birthday calls from both of us, the drunken accusatory calls from her, and the occasional call from her to share the latest piece of news or gossip. My mom loved to recount horror stories. Maybe they were her way of making her life seem like it was not that bad in comparison. When she called to tell me she had some bad news, I knew this call was different from the usual run of the mill ones. Her voice sounded sober, and scared, and very far away. This time the horror story she shared was her own. She told me she had breast cancer and they were going to do a mastectomy followed by chemotherapy. I think most daughters who have just been told their mother has breast cancer would be devastated, or at least extremely upset. I felt no compassion. The judgemental and unforgiving parts of me thought cancer was payback for the many hurtful things she had done to others in her life. I did not even shed a tear. I vaguely remember delivering some platitude, not unlike the birthday and Mother's Day cards I usually sent. I think I told her everything would be fine. When I write about this now I am appalled by how much I closed off my heart. But I had nothing to give back then. I was still too full of anger. Anger was not something that could be expressed when I was a child and I was still like that child when interacting with my mother. Our past was simmering just below the surface between us. We never spoke about it. Yet, what was not spoken loomed unseen and energetically larger than life between us. I had no interest in trying to close that gap then. Forgiveness was not even on the radar.

Tools for Transformation

- *Do you have a relationship in your life that feels heavy with things that have not been spoken? Is it possible for you to open up the lines of communication in some way? If not, can you open your heart and send loving energy to that person?*

- *Are there areas of your life where anger might be standing in the way of forgiveness? What might lie beneath your anger?*

8. The Birth of My First Daughter

"Hush little baby, don't say a word, Mama's gonna buy you a mockingbird.
If that mockingbird don't sing, Mama's gonna buy you a diamond ring.
If that diamond ring turns brass, Mama's gonna buy you a looking glass.
If that looking glass gets broke, Mama's gonna buy you a billy goat.
If that billy goat won't pull, Mama's gonna buy you a cart and bull.
If that cart and bull turn over, Mama's gonna buy you a dog named Rover.
If that dog named Rover won't bark,
Mama's gonna buy you a horse and cart.
If that horse and cart fall down, you'll still be the sweetest little baby in town."

Hush Little Baby—A traditional lullaby

MY MOTHER WAS NOT INVITED to be there after I gave birth to her first grandchild. I could not rely on her being sober. The last thing I wanted to do was deal with a drunk at the same time as I was recovering from giving birth and trying to look after a new baby. On a conscious level that was true. If I were to tell the whole truth I would also need to acknowledge I was subconsciously trying to punish her for all the times she had not been there for me as a child. Not that I saw that back then. I felt I was justified in my decision. I only wanted my husband with me at the hospital.

Our beautiful baby girl was born on the Saturday of Easter weekend. My water broke at 6:30 in the morning the day before my due date. We had the hospital bag packed and ready to go for a couple of weeks. When the contractions got more regular and closer together we got in the car and headed to the hospital. It was not far away but the trip felt long. My senses were heightened and every detail was vivid. I remember the coat I wore, the car we were in, and the drive. When the highway sign for the hospital finally appeared I was relieved. The pain from the contractions was not intense yet, but I was afraid. I had not given birth before and did not know exactly what to expect. We had gone to pre-natal classes and hoped for natural childbirth, but we also knew every birth is different. My mom had not really told me much about her birthing experiences. The only thing she shared was that her mother told her giving birth was the most pain she would ever feel.

When we got to the hospital the nurses discovered meconium in my amniotic fluid. They told me that meant the baby had a bowel movement and might be in distress. Plans for natural childbirth went out the window as they hooked the baby and me up to machines to monitor our heartbeats. This meant I was flat on my back during labour. Not a position conducive to helping the birth progress. After several hours of labour they gave me an epidural. By the time I was well into the pushing stage I had been in labour almost 12 hours. The heart monitor began to indicate the baby was going into distress. There was a flurry of doctors and nurses around me. I was overwhelmed and scared. They immediately began to prep me for surgery. They said they were going to attempt a forceps delivery, but if that did not work they would do a Caesarean section. They also told me they had a respiratory specialist waiting on standby. As soon as the baby was born they were going to take it away and suction the meconium out of its throat and breathing passages before it cried. Inhaling the meconium could cause respiratory problems for the baby. When they used the forceps they just got the baby turned and she was born very quickly. As soon as her head was out she began screaming. So much for getting the meconium suctioned out before she cried. They took her away and removed all the meconium they could. Then they kept her for a while to watch her carefully.

It was 8:05 pm when Allison made her entrance into the world. By 9:00 pm she was back with me breastfeeding. I was so relieved and grateful she was okay. She was perfect with her dark hair, olive skin, and intense eyes. She looked a lot like her father. I could hardly believe this baby was ours. During the nine months I carried her inside of me I thought she might be a boy but I wondered if she would be a girl. I wondered what she would look like. I loved her before I met her. Now after the long wait, here she was. The love I had for her before I met her transformed to a love I had never known. It was a fierce love that brought up every protective instinct I had. I knew, without question, I would give my life for this little soul. I vowed I would parent differently from my mother. I made up my mind I would do everything with a girl baby I would have done with a boy. Everything about Allison mesmerised me. Her perfectly formed hands and feet and her tiny fingernails. I used to watch her little chest rise and fall with each breath and stand in awe of this being who had chosen me to be her mother. There are some beautiful pictures of her first days at the hospital. One is of her sleeping peacefully in her bassinet. She looks like an angel in human form. My other favourite is of her and her father. He is sitting in a chair beside my hospital bed holding Allison shortly after she was born. The look on his face definitely shines with love at first sight.

The after effects of the labour, epidural, mid-forceps delivery, and subsequent surgical repairs took a lot out of me physically. I was not able to stand for very long before I would begin to pass out. The baby and I ended up staying in the hospital for three days. Her dad did all of her diaper changes for those first few days. I was sad I could not do more. I felt somehow less than, because I was not physically able to look after my own daughter. The babies were kept in the hospital nursery at night so the moms could get some rest. They were brought to their moms for feeding. Allison was one of the first babies they brought. She was not shy about letting the nurses know she was hungry! I could hear her crying all the way down the hall. If the nurses waited too long Allison would wake up all the other babies in the nursery with her demands to be fed. I remember thinking this little girl would go far in the world because she knew how to get what she needed. I felt lulled into a sense of security while we were in the hospital. If something went wrong I felt confident they would be able to handle it.

Wanting to Do it Differently From the Generations Before Me

Three days after Allison was born we loaded the flowers and gifts into our vehicle. We put our baby into her car seat for the first time so she could make her trip home safely. I felt like I was in a foreign land again. My life had changed so vastly in just three days. I went from a woman expecting a baby to a mother completely responsible 24 hours a day for this precious living being that was gifted to me. I was in awe, bewilderment, and overwhelm all at the same time. I had chosen to not have my mother by my side through any of it.

My husband took two weeks off work so he could be home to help take care of the baby in the first few weeks of her life. I am very grateful that he did. He was a big help. He made the meals, helped clean up, and did more than his share of diaper changes. He would go and get Allison and bring her to me for her feedings in the middle of the night. Within less than a month she was beginning to sleep through the night. Allison's dad carried her around like a football on his arm. The 'football hold' and his willingness to walk around with her when she needed soothing really helped us begin to settle into our new life. He had much more confidence to try new things with her than I did. I would find something that worked and then would not want to deviate from it. I wanted so much to be a good mother. I learned what *not to do* from my own mother. But I did not really have a role model for what *to do*.

Our baby grew in leaps and bounds. She was a serious baby most of the time. But she also had a smile that lit up her whole face. My days revolved around her schedule. When she napped I tried to get some rest and when she was up we spent our time together. She showed me where some of the gaps were in my own upbringing. I found it was a challenge for me to play with her because I did not remember playing much as a child. Letting her express what she needed to express without trying to shut her down was another hurdle. There was also a small part of me that was beginning to think that the incredible amount of love I had for my child must have also been present somewhere in my mother, for me. If it was there at one time, I wondered where it had gone. My daughter was showing me it was impossible to not love your own child. So, what were the barriers inside of my mother that prevented her from showing love to me? Maybe she loved me with everything she had, and it was not the way I needed and wanted to be loved. Perhaps the self-loathing she lived with every day blocked the love from coming through. Or maybe her love was there and my anger prevented me from seeing it. I was beginning to open up enough to question the relationship between my mother and me, but my days were so busy with the baby I did not yet have a lot of time to search for the answers.

There was much advice handed to me during my pregnancy and after Allison was born. Everyone seemed to be an expert in raising children. Especially those people who never had any. The best piece of advice and one of the few I followed came from the wife of one of the managers I used to work with. He was retiring shortly before I was starting my maternity leave. All of the managers and their spouses went out for dinner to celebrate. I ended up seated beside his wife. What she said to me has stayed with me always. She told me she raised five children. When her children were grown someone asked her youngest daughter what she remembered most about her childhood. The daughter's response was that she remembered the house was always clean. My new friend told me it broke her heart to hear this. She said it was true. In her day, being a good housewife meant that taking care of the house came first. Everything needed to be shiny, clean, and organised. Once that was taken care of, and only then, could time be spent with the kids. So her children did not remember having fun; they remembered having a clean house. Her words of wisdom were that the house would wait and my time would be better spent with my children.

The Façade of the Happy Family Begins to Crack

'Spending time with my child is a priority' became a motto I lived by. Unfortunately, my husband's views were not the same on the matter. He liked a neat and tidy house and he could not understand what I did with my time all day. When he came home after work to a house that was upside down he was not happy. This was a disagreement that remained unresolved throughout our whole relationship. To the outside world we looked like the perfect happy family. In those days appearances were everything to both of us.

When Allison was a couple of months old her father was offered a new job. It would mean moving to Toronto. If he did not accept the job offer he would not be able to be promoted to the next level of management and his career would come to a standstill. The catch was the cost of living was much higher in Toronto and it was going to cost us $130,000 more for a house that was comparable to what we were presently living in. He accepted the new job and began flying to Toronto every Monday morning and flying home on Friday night. This meant I was alone all week with the demands of a very young baby. All of our carefully laid plans were falling apart. We were going from no mortgage to a $130,000 mortgage on one salary, and we would be a 40 minute drive from my mother. Allison was six months old when we packed up our life and headed to Toronto.

Being in close proximity to my family turned out to be a mixed blessing. The good part was I loved being able to see my brothers more often. I really missed them. It was great to get together with them at family functions, and Allison loved her uncles. Neither of them was married, or had children, and they were wonderful with her. The not-so-good part was being that close to my mother meant I would need to set some boundaries with her around alcohol. She would not be able to spend time with Allison alone if she was drinking. To my amazement, she never crossed that line. She was head over heels in love with her granddaughter. She was available for Allison like she had never been available for me as a child. She got right down in the sandbox with her to build sand castles. She spent hours at the mall with Allison paying for her to go on all the kiddie rides. Allison could make a mess and eat as many cookies as she wanted at Grandma's house. I sometimes think my mother willed herself to stay alive long enough to have time with her grandchildren. If felt to me like she thought this was her last chance at the whole mothering thing and she was desperate to get it right this time. I watched the two of them together with mixed emotions. Delight that my mother had such capacity for love for my daughter and envious that she was not able to offer the same to me when I was a child. My mom may not have done a very good job as a mother but she made up for it in her role as grandmother. She sang to Allison and read her stories. She pushed Allison in the swing in her backyard for as long as Allison wanted to swing. There was nothing else more pressing that was calling her. I think in some small way she may have been trying to reach out to me through what was nearest and dearest to me. Consequently, my mother and I began to spend more time together, connected through the heart of my daughter.

I tried to follow my intuition and go with what felt right to me in raising my daughter. I found this was not an easy thing to do. I did not realise how much pressure there would be to conform to existing authoritarian methods of child rearing. This pressure came from all sides. From my spouse, my mother, and society. It became a source of conflict between my husband and me. He and his mother thought we should let the baby cry herself to sleep and that picking her up too often would spoil her. It felt very wrong to me to not comfort a crying baby. The thought of leaving her alone to cry in her crib was way too reminiscent of my childhood and something I was not prepared to do. I vowed I would not abuse my child like I was abused. I still used spanking as a form of discipline though. I did not use wooden spoons or kettle cords or backhands like my mother had done, and so I thought that made it all right.

It soon became evident my husband and I could not afford a $130,000 mortgage on one salary and I wept at the thought of going back to work and putting our baby in daycare. My husband did not necessarily understand my desire to stay at home with Allison but he tolerated it. We made the decision to sell our home and buy a smaller one in the same town. I loved the new house. It was the first house where I was given carte blanche to decorate any way I wanted. Previous houses were kept in neutral builder's beige because my husband was transferred fairly often with work. Resale was kept in mind with each house purchase. This house was one we planned to live in for a long time. It was small and cozy. Most people who came to visit said it felt warmer than our previous homes. My husband did not view it that way. One night he made the comment that he was not happy with his life. He said he was not anywhere near where he expected to be at his age. Somehow he looked at the downsizing of our house as a commentary on his ability to provide for his family. He felt like he had failed.

It turned out my husband and I had lots of differing thoughts on how life should be lived. Not discussing them before we got married did nothing to keep them from coming up now. The added stress of adjusting to life with a baby and lack of sleep were the fuel. Financial worry was the spark that started the fire. But neither one of us talked about what was bothering us. Instead, we used passive aggressive ways to let each other know we were upset. He spent more money, got drunk occasionally, and had more angry outbursts about seemingly insignificant things. I gained weight, developed a debilitating case of premenstrual syndrome (PMS), and became less and less interested in sex. Our problems never had a chance of being resolved because neither one of us was willing to bring them to the table.

The conflict that we did not acknowledge as conflict, and the distance in our relationship increased. All of this coincided with Allison entering her terrible twos. Her struggle for independence and her constant limit testing collided head on with my worry about my marriage. I found myself using spanking more and more as a form of discipline. I was not comfortable with this, but I did not know what else to do. It got to the point where it felt like the spankings were more for my benefit than for hers. I worried I would cross the line into physical abuse. So I went to talk to my family doctor. She gave me some recommendations to deal with the PMS. She also reassured me that the fact I was questioning myself around the spanking meant I would not cross the line with it. I was not so sure. In the heat of the moment, no matter what my best intentions were, I resorted to what I experienced as a child: corporal punishment.

Tools for Transformation

- *When life does not turn out as you expected how do you respond?*

- *What do you do with external pressure to do something that does not fit with your values?*

- *What are your values? (See the Values List in the Resource Section at the end of the book.) Make a list and hold onto it. We will look at values in more depth in Chapter 11.*

- *Have you ever found yourself reacting in situations and wondering where the reaction came from? Can you trace any of these reactive patterns to your childhood? Are you willing to begin to look at new ways of responding to old triggers? We will talk more about this in Part III of the book.*

The Birth of My First Daughter

9. The Birth of My Second Daughter

"Lavender's blue, dilly dilly, lavender's green.
When you are king, dilly dilly, I shall be queen.
Who told you so, dilly dilly, who told you so?
'Twas my own heart, dilly dilly, that told me so."

17ᵗʰ Century English Folk Song & Nursery Rhyme

A FEW MONTHS AFTER ALLISON'S SECOND BIRTHDAY I discovered I was expecting another baby. The pregnancy came as a bit of a surprise. We talked about having a second child but had not really made any definite plans yet. My husband was an only child and enjoyed it for the most part. He had five cousins he grew up in close contact with. In contrast to the hectic pace of their home I believe he enjoyed his quiet alone time with his mom and dad. He could not relate to what it would be like to have siblings because he did not have any. I, on the other hand, could not imagine growing up without brothers and/or sisters. Even though my brothers and I fought a lot with each other when we were kids, we also protected each other. Now that we were adults we really loved each other. I attributed the childhood conflict between my brothers and me to how close we were in age. I felt none of us got our needs met because we were all clamouring for attention at the same time. I thought three years between children would be good timing. It would allow our first child to have lots of individual time with us before the next child came along.

I felt irritable and nauseous for several weeks and could not figure out why. I had my period so I did not think about being pregnant. But when my period ended and I still had breast tenderness and some nausea I decided to try a home pregnancy test. The result was positive. I wondered if it was a false positive as I had not heard of anyone having a period at the beginning of a pregnancy. I wondered if I might be miscarrying. I went to our family doctor and did a pregnancy test there. The results came back positive. I called my husband at work to let him know. Even though the news was unexpected, we both looked forward to the new baby. I really liked the idea of having more than one child. I hoped they would grow to love each other as much as my brothers and I had. My only concern was would I be able to love this second baby as much as I loved Allison?

Even though I was not working outside of my home, I was busy with a two year old and getting time to rest was a challenge. I was much more tired this time. I tried to rest when Allison went down for her afternoon nap each day. We began transitioning Allison out of her crib and into a 'big girl bed' quite a while before the new baby's due date, so she would not feel displaced. Allison and I began to travel once a week to visit my mother. My mom seemed to have more energy than I did. She played with Allison a lot while I sat and watched. It was a relief to share some of the demands of a two year old with someone else.

My pregnancy went well and the time passed quickly. Before I knew it my due date had almost arrived. The day before it, I started getting cramps at 4:00 am. My mucous plug came away at 8:00 am but my water had not broken. My husband had gone to work, so I called my mom to come and stay with Allison and me. Her neighbour drove her down around lunch time. By 2:30 pm my contractions were five minutes apart. My husband came home from work and we headed to the hospital at 3:30 pm. My mom stayed to look after Allison. I was three centimetres dilated. By 7:00 pm I was only four centimetres dilated. They broke my water hoping to move my labour along to the next stage. All it did was make the labour pains worse. They tried laughing gas (nitrous oxide) to relax me but it did not work. I was starting to panic. By 8:50 pm I asked for a shot of Demerol. Our daughter Laken was born at 9:08 pm. Her dad headed off to go curling with his team after he made sure the baby and I were fine. Because Laken was born so soon after the Demerol, quite a bit of it was still in her system. As a result she was a very quiet baby for a few days. I had to wake her to breastfeed. Within two days she found her lungs and her appetite. She was the complete opposite to her sister in many ways. Laken had fair skin and fair hair. As much as Allison resembled her father, Laken was almost an exact likeness of me. We spent three days in the hospital. I only had a few stitches this time and my recovery was much faster. I was able to get up and around quickly after the birth. My husband brought Allison and my mom to the hospital to visit the new baby. Allison seemed quite enthralled. I need not have worried about whether I would love the second baby as much as the first. I did. When it comes to children, I am amazed by the capacity for love in a mother's heart.

My mom had somewhat of a different reaction to Laken. Laken looked like me and I looked very much like my father. Even Laken's hands were shaped like my dad's. My mom remarked on how Laken's pinkie finger had the same crook in it as my dad's and mine. I had not noticed it until my mom pointed it out. Looking at Laken was a constant reminder of my dad. It was a beautiful remembrance for me, but it brought up difficult memories for my mom.

I Have Been Promoted to My Level of Incompetence

After Allison was born, I was still masking my doubts and putting on a brave front. I was able to keep it all together. To the outside world it looked like we were happily married. We had a beautiful home and family. One method of self-preservation I learned growing up in an alcoholic family was control. My life as a child was chaotic and totally out of my control. As I grew older my way of dealing with that was to try to control everything around me. Keeping it together, at all costs, was part of the whole control package. With the birth of my second child the illusion of control began to slip through my fingers and I could not keep it all together anymore.

Around age 30 seems to be a turning point for many people. Previous emotional stuff we think we have buried begins to poke its head up to be looked at. Maybe it is because we are beginning to have the emotional maturity to deal with it by then. Maybe life has worn us down enough that fatigue makes it more difficult to hold things inside. Or maybe it is our soul's way of telling us this is the time in our journey when we chose to move on to the next phase of our evolution. There is no way to go around or jump over what is weighing us down. The only way to the other side is through.

Whatever the reason, I was no exception. I was 32 when Laken was born. I felt stirrings of emotional unrest after Allison's birth but was able to keep the lid on them. Baby number two blew the lid sky high. Unlike her sister, Laken woke several times during the night until she was close to a year old. As much as my husband tried to get me to let her cry herself to sleep, I refused to do it. When I would go and pick her up from her crib, she would have her little knees drawn up to her tummy. She was having gastro-intestinal distress and the only thing that seemed to soothe her was being rocked or walked for a while until the gas passed. When she was not in pain, she was a happy baby. One of the ways I could get her to laugh was to sing her the lullaby *Lavender's Blue* and hold her over my head for the "dilly, dilly" verse.

The baby novelty seemed to have worn off for my husband after our first child. Where he had been quite involved from day one with Allison, he barely picked Laken up until she was close to two months old. The two weeks he took off work after Allison was born to help me dwindled to a couple of days with Laken. He was helping out with Allison where he could in the evenings after he got home from work. If Allison got up in the middle of the night he would tend to her. But he did not focus much time or attention on Laken. He said she was a baby and would not know the difference. She did. So did I. Perhaps he had good reasons for his absence. I really did not care what the reasons were. I needed his help. As was the pattern in our family, I did not ask him for it. I expected him to read my mind and know what I needed. I was having misgivings about my marriage and I was not taking care of myself physically, emotionally, mentally, or spiritually. My well ran dry and I had nothing left to give. I was exhausted all the time. Resentment did not make a good bed fellow and making love dropped to the bottom of my priority list. Our sex life was at an all-time low. Having two children was more than twice the work of having one. There was not just the fatigue to deal with, but sibling rivalry as well. As much as Allison was intrigued by her little sister, she was not thrilled with giving up her role as the only child. Having mom and dad's attention cut by more than half was not sitting well with her. I would turn my back for a moment and the baby would be screaming because Allison pinched or bit her. Laken was born just six weeks before Allison's third birthday. I discovered the terrible twos had nothing on the trying threes!

Verbally Abusing My First Daughter

I tried not to spank Allison as much and began using a time-out chair instead. But there were still times when I lost it and in the heat of the moment I would give her a swat on the behind. The swats were usually a knee-jerk reaction to Allison hitting her sister. At the time I did not see the irony in hitting my child in order to teach her to not hit someone else. I do not know when I crossed the line into verbal abuse. Maybe I had been doing that all along and just never noticed it. Somewhere in the back of my mind I think I justified yelling as less damaging than spanking.

There were often nights I got little sleep. The days after those nights would be the worst. I had little patience and Allison seemed to pick up energetically on my inner turmoil. We would feed off of each other and the tension would spiral higher and higher. Eventually she would do or say something that pushed one of my hidden emotional buttons and I would lose my temper.

There was not anything special about the day when I made up my mind to do something different. It was a day like every other day, where I woke up feeling tired, frustrated, and overwhelmed. Despite my vows to parent differently from the generations before me, I found I was becoming my mother. When I was angry, I subconsciously allowed the reptilian part of my brain to take over. I exhibited the parenting behaviour I learned at the hands of my mother. I did what I knew, what the neural pathways laid down in my brain from childhood programming directed me to do. It may not have been functional but it was familiar. I felt like a failure and I hated myself for it.

I do not remember exactly what Allison had done, or not done, to set me off. Whatever it was, I used it as an excuse to vent all of my frustration on her. We were standing in the hallway of the pantry just off the kitchen. She was facing me as I stood over her screaming at the top of my lungs. It was almost as if I had left my body and some menacing shrew had inhabited it. Allison stood frozen on the spot looking up at me. Something made me look into her three-year-old eyes. What I saw there was absolute terror. That terror sparked a remembrance in me of what it felt like to be the child target of an adult's rage, to watch the face of the person you love most in the world contort with such fury that it is almost unrecognizable, and to fear for your life because you did not know what might come next. Her eyes reflected my childhood pain and without a word she touched my soul. In that moment a switch flipped inside of me. I did not want my children to fear me. I wanted a relationship with them built on safety, love, trust, and respect. What the hell had I been doing? I made a conscious choice in the kitchen that day. I told myself, "The abuse stops here." I did not want this passed on to another generation. I knew there had to be a way to change things, even if I did not yet know how. That choice was pivotal in altering the course of my and my family's future.

Going to Parenting Classes

As much as I tried to make changes on my own, I slipped up often. I was beginning to understand parenting is one of the most challenging and important jobs in the world. And it is the one with the least training. We are expected to know what to do just because we have the biological capability to produce a child. We receive more training to drive a car, an inanimate object that will end up being tossed on the scrap heap after a few years. Our children are with us for life, if we are very lucky, and they do not come with instruction manuals. I was stumped about the whole parenting thing. I did not have good role models in this area. Even though I was now aware I could be a better parent, I still was not doing better at it consistently.

I was reading our local paper one day and came across an ad for parenting classes that were being offered in my community. There was an unwritten rule in my family about not airing your dirty laundry in public. I allowed my ego to keep me hung up on that excuse for a while. Taking parenting classes would be like admitting to the world I did not know what I was doing. Some childhood fears came up about possibly having my children taken away from me if I admitted I was challenged as a parent. In the end I knew my goal of not repeating the past was more important than my fear and I registered for the class.

I learned a great many things in that class. First of all I was not alone. There were several of us there. All of these people were just like me. They found what they were doing was not working and they were looking for a better way. There were lots of tips and tools and practice sessions in class. It was based on Dr. Thomas Gordon's *Parent Effectiveness Training* material. The text and workbook claimed this was a tested new way to raise responsible children. That was exactly what I wanted. I did not want to raise children who were obedient out of fear, as I was. I wanted to raise children who could think for themselves and be motivated by love. I wanted discipline to be about inspiring them to live life more effectively, not about punishing and shaming them. The classes were filled with lots of ideas that were outside my realm of parenting experience and they opened up a whole new world for me.

Somewhere in that process I learned to begin to let go of my impossible standard of being a perfect mother. The pendulum of learning had swung from the extremes of my mother's 'bad mothering' to my attempt at 'perfect mothering' and was beginning to settle at a more balanced place of 'good enough mothering'. I was acknowledging my humanness in the whole process. And learning that modelling the behaviour I was looking for in my children spoke much louder than my words ever would. The key was to stay in my integrity. When I missed the mark I felt it in my gut. Then, instead of beating myself up mentally about it, I would apologise to my children and make a concentrated effort to do better the next time. To my knowledge, mine were the first adult apologies given to the children in my extended family.

Seeking Counselling

Without the outlet of venting my anger on my children, more and more of my unhealed emotional baggage began to rise to the surface. It was stored inside of me for 32 years and now it had nowhere to go. I was like a volcano, lots going on underneath the surface that was invisible to the naked eye, with the odd angry flare up every now and again. But, for the most part, the pressure was contained within me. I was afraid if I started to release it I would not be able to control the eruption, that I would hurt people, and ultimately my ego believed I would perish.

The energy required to keep the tide of emotions submerged was exhausting me. I began to sink into a depression. That scared me more than anything else. I wondered if I was heading down the same path as my father. The doctors diagnosed his as clinical depression. I did not know exactly what that meant, but I certainly did not want to travel the lonely road he had.

I headed back to my family doctor. Once again she reassured me. She said if I was prone to clinical depression it would have manifested in my life much younger than 32. She gave me a prescription for Prozac. I tried that for a while but I was flat-lined emotionally. I was not feeling the lows anymore, but I also was not feeling the highs. The colours in my world blended into a sea of grey. I was barely treading water. I really did not care one way or the other about much of anything. This was not how I wanted to live. After another visit to the doctor to get off of Prozac, she recommended I see a counsellor. Going for counselling was even more taboo in my family than going to parenting classes was. There was still such a stigma around it. I did not want to be thought of as crazy. At first I did not tell anyone other than my husband that I was going. He did not really understand why I wanted to go, but he told me to do what I thought I needed to do. When I eventually told my brothers I was going for counselling my youngest brother told me I was causing my own problems. That some things were better left alone. I did not tell my mom I was going.

Tools for Transformation

- *Are you able to ask for what you need? Do you expect others to read your mind? Make a list of 3 things that you are stressed about. Then make a list of 10 sources of support you can call on. Within the next week choose one of the things from your list of stressors and ask someone from your list of sources of support for help with it. The first person or organisation you ask may or may not be able to help. This is not a commentary on whether or not you are deserving of help. You are. If the first person or organisation you ask is unavailable, go on to the next on your list. Keep asking until you have success.*

- *Are there areas of your life where you do not know what to do, but think you should know? We all learn different things at different points in our life. It takes most of us several lifetimes to master certain concepts. You are entitled to the time it takes to learn. Pick an area of your life that is not working the way you would like it to and open yourself up to the possibility of seeking knowledge in that area. We are all students and teachers in life. What you need to learn, someone else is here to teach, and vice versa. There will be a person, book, song, an organisation, or a workshop that will help you on your way. What step could you take to gain knowledge and experience in an area of interest to you?*

- *Is striving for perfection keeping you stuck? Can you reframe any thoughts you might have of being a 'perfect anything' and allow yourself to dance with the possibility of being a 'good enough anything'? Can you allow for, and honour your humanness as you continue to learn and grow?*

10. My Dark Night of the Soul

"The Dark Night of the Soul—between no longer and not yet."

Joan Borysenko

I FELT SELFISH FOR WANTING MORE than life was currently offering me. I had a husband, a nice home, and beautiful children I adored. I had loving brothers and many wonderful friends. What more could I possibly ask for? Why could I not be happy with what I had? The truth was I did not have an answer to those questions. Continuing to ask "why?" was not helping. It just gave the harsh judge inside of me more fuel. I was digging myself a deep hole with my continuous cycle of self-recrimination. Instead of acknowledging what I was feeling, I was trying to use my intellect to figure it out. I was looking for an explanation and an external solution to make the pain inside go away. It was not bringing me any closer to happiness.

Mustering up the courage to go for counselling was a long drawn out process. I knew what I could remember of my past, and the shape I was in now. Panic set in with thoughts that counselling might dredge up repressed memories I would not be able to handle. The day came when the hole I was digging for myself was so deep I feared I would bury myself alive. I called for a counselling appointment.

I experienced a mixed bag of emotions during the first meeting with the counsellor. I felt some relief that I was finally doing something about my unrest. I was scared of the unknown. I felt sick to my stomach because I was going against my family's rules of silence about the past. I did not even reveal what was going on inside of me to the people who were closest to me. How would I be able to do that with a perfect stranger? What if he could not help me? Oh my God, what if the counsellor could not help me? It felt like this was my last resort. If counselling failed, and I was destined to continue living this life of quiet desperation, I did not know what I would do.

The first appointment went okay. He was kind and soft spoken. I began to relax a little. After a few appointments, I started to learn a little more about what was involved in counselling. The counsellor was not there to fix me. He was there as my guide as I explored my inner resources and learned how to help myself. We only had a couple of sessions together when he zeroed in on what he called one of my core issues, that of being an adult child of an alcoholic (ACOA). This was not a term I had heard before. There was an eight week ACOA group being led by a colleague of his that was starting up in a few weeks. He suggested I might want to consider joining it. Seeing a counsellor was one thing, but the thought of talking about my deepest feelings in a group of strangers was quite another. It took everything in me to register for the group. But the higher part of me knew that was where I needed to be. So I dragged myself, silently kicking and screaming, to the first group session.

It was comforting to discover a name for the things I was experiencing. I felt some days like I was losing my mind. But apparently there were many ACOAs out there having a similar experience. I felt less alone knowing we had developed common coping strategies. We shared characteristics like: guessing at what normal was because we had not experienced it when we were kids, judging ourselves mercilessly, taking ourselves and life way too seriously, being hyper-vigilant and unable to have fun, experiencing difficulty navigating intimate relationships, and blaming ourselves for the chaos that was our family life, to name a few. Any one of these things would be a challenge. But the toxic mixture of all of them was often debilitating. No wonder I was struggling.

Three pivotal things happened in the group that began to open my eyes to a new perception of my world. The first was that we did the *Myers-Briggs Type Indicator* test, which was basically a personality type assessment questionnaire. We answered the 88 questions and then the questionnaires were sent out to a lady who was experienced in interpreting the answers. The questions helped to distinguish between two different extremes in four different categories. Our answers in the first category placed us somewhere on the scale between introvert and extravert. The next two categories looked at whether we used sensing or intuition more, and whether we tended toward thinking or feeling. Lastly, did we use more judging or perceiving in our lifestyle? She brought the questionnaires back to our next group meeting with our results. One of the first questions she asked was, "Who is Denise?" I wanted a hole to open up in the floor so I could drop into it and out of sight. I was afraid my answers to the questions indicated I was irreparably damaged. She told me I was the first person in all the years she had been giving these tests whose answers in the introvert/extravert category were all on the introvert side of the scale. She said she could only imagine what a challenge it was for me to be in a group for counselling. She also acknowledged that my level of commitment to my healing must have been extremely high to venture into a group setting. I breathed a sigh of relief. Somebody finally understood me and told me I was okay. The test showed me some of my personality qualities were intrinsic. I used to assume I was defective. I thought if I could find ways to change all the things that were wrong with me I could be happy. This kind of thinking turned me into a square peg trying to fit myself into a round hole. The test showed me there were some things that were innate to my personality and those things were not wrong. They contributed to my uniqueness. I began to understand why certain things were challenging for me. Which did not mean they were impossible. For instance, I was always going to be an introvert, but I could choose to go outside of my comfort zone when I was called to. It was not necessary to change the essence of who I was to be okay.

The second thing that impacted me in a big way was, as a group we used John Bradshaw's book *Homecoming: Reclaiming and Championing Your Inner Child*, as a study guide. We began to work our way through the chapters and exercises in the book. I had not heard the term 'inner child' before. But, as I tried some of the exercises in the book, I began to sense the truth of that child part inside of me. She had been crying out for a long time. My mother was the first to have taken on the role of silencing that child. As I grew older, I internalised the voice of her verbal abuse into my own inner critic. I no longer needed my mother to silence my inner child. I became adept at doing it myself. This little girl in me had a lot to express, although I was having difficulty listening. During the course of the ACOA group, PBS aired a John Bradshaw special on the *Homecoming*. I taped it and watched it several times. Almost everything he talked about spoke directly to my heart. I was so excited to have 'expert' confirmation of all that was going on inside of me. I asked my husband if he would sit down and watch some of the key parts with me. His comment after watching was this was probably the latest self-help guru. In a few months there would be someone else who would come along to debunk this theory and present a completely different one. I was crushed. I had tentatively reached out to him for some understanding and support in my journey into the depths of who I was. My first gesture of sharing that tender part inside of me with my husband was met with disqualification. I decided not to risk making myself vulnerable with him again.

The last pivotal piece came for me when the counsellor who was facilitating the group took me aside after one of the group sessions. She asked if I had ever considered being a counsellor. She said I had a natural gift for it and that the other members of the group already looked to me as a leader and a role model. I considered going into counselling in high school. But back then I thought about the fact that kids whom I might counsel would end up going back into their dysfunctional family homes. At the time I did not see how counselling could have any lasting impact in those kinds of circumstances. I did not know how I could counsel someone and then not take home all of their angst with me at the end of the day. Now, I was at a point where I knew even the smallest gesture could have a huge impact in the life of another. Through the ACOA group I was beginning to learn about boundaries and I was also getting a glimpse of my potential. I thanked the facilitator for her kind words and I filed the idea of being a counsellor away in my mind.

As we progressed through the book, other exercises, and group discussions, I began to see my dad's role in my childhood abuse. Even though he never laid a hand on me, he had not done anything to stop my mother from abusing me. I do not know if he was unaware of the abuse, if he turned a blind eye to it to avoid conflict with my mother, or if he felt powerless to intervene. The reason did not really matter because the end result was the same. The children in our family were left to fend for themselves. Taking my dad off the pedestal I had him on since I was a child was one of the hardest things I ever had to do. In my mind he was one of the only good constants I had to hang onto. He was my rock. Being able to tell myself that at least my dad had not abused me, helped me feel some part of me was lovable. It was like being able to hold onto a branch on the side of the river as the rushing current was trying to sweep me along and over the waterfall. With this new insight about my dad, that branch snapped and I was tossed about in the current. I was heading for the waterfall and I had nothing recognizable to stop my plunge.

The hurt and pain I had stored since I was a child was being dislodged. What was buried, I buried deep. As it resurfaced, it brought with it unresolved emotional memories from my childhood. It also brought up the muck and sludge the memories were buried in. What was rising up was like bile in my throat. But I would not allow myself to purge it. The little girl inside of me was deathly afraid. Attending the ACOA group released some of the poison from my past. The problem was I did not know of a way, or even that there was a need, to move it out of my body somehow.

The darkest part of my life occurred while I was attending the group, and for a long while after. I felt heaviness in my body all the time. I cried a lot and I felt like I was carrying around a lead weight on my chest. I hit my rock bottom. Many doors to knowledge were opened for me. But many doors to the unknown opened unbidden simultaneously. I had a pretty good idea of what I was leaving behind, but no idea of where I was headed to. I felt like I was attempting a high-wire act for the first time. Too afraid to let go of the old rope I was holding onto in order to grab the new rope that was swinging toward me. Grabbing the new rope would require a split second in mid-air where I was not hanging onto anything at all. I did not remember that there was a support net to catch me if I fell. It was a scary and a lonely place to be. I was frozen in the pain from my past and allowing it to cast shadows on my present and plant seeds of darkness for my future. I was living everywhere but in my body in the present moment.

Once the ACOA group was finished, my main source of support for the healing journey I had begun was finished too. My husband had not really expressed an interest in what I was doing. He just hoped I would get back to 'normal' soon. I had not told any of my friends I was going for counselling, so I felt like I could not go to them for help. My family really did not want to hear about it either. I think in some ways I may have been threatening people's equilibrium. If I changed, how would that affect them? As much as I wanted my life to be different I feared change too. I may not have liked what was going on in my life, but at least it was familiar and I was able to handle it in the past. The uncharted territory of the unknown tested my belief in myself.

I carried on in the other routines of life. For all intents and purposes it appeared things were going okay. I lived day to day, pulling myself out of bed every morning to tend to my two beautiful children. I dropped, exhausted in to bed every night. I got myself a part-time job on evenings and weekends to help support us financially and that helped me feel better for a while. When the good feelings from that wore off, I made an attempt to exercise and watch my food intake. I got myself down to a healthy weight and that gave me a boost for a short time. Losing the weight gave me more energy and I felt better about myself, but it still was not enough.

The external solutions I was seeking to quell the anxiety in me were all only temporary. As one wore off, the search for the next would begin. I kept thinking surely this next one would be the permanent solution to my problems. I did not know at the time that healing would involve working with and balancing the physical, emotional, mental, and spiritual parts of me. I was not even aware I had that many layers. I also did not yet know that the healing would have to come from within. There was nothing outside of me that was going to bring me peace.

Tools for Transformation

- *Can you identify times when you have sought external sources of happiness? Did they bring you lasting peace?*

- *Have you heard the voice of the higher part of you speaking to you sometimes? How often do you listen to it?*

- *Are there times when you feel like you have lost your mind? Was it necessarily a bad thing, or did it give you an opportunity to drop into your heart and feel your feelings?*

- *Identify three pivotal moments in your life and how they have changed the trajectory of your journey.*

- *What are the intrinsic parts of you (the qualities you were born with)? Are you accepting of them? Which of these parts do you think make you uniquely you?*

- *Do you have an inner critic? Whose recriminating voices have you internalised (more on this in Chapter 20)? Are they speaking the truth about you? Do their messages serve your highest good?*

- *Have you met your amazing inner child? Find a picture of yourself as a child and make several photocopies of it. Put these copies in places where you are going to see them often (i.e. the fridge, bathroom mirror, your desk, your computer monitor, the dashboard of your car, etc.). They will remind you of that tender part inside of you that holds lots of wisdom and the key to your heart. As you begin to champion your inner child, be discerning about whom you share her/him with. People who have not done their own inner child work will not likely be able to support you in doing yours. As you begin to build trust with this little person you do not want to enlist the help of an adult who is going to stomp on that new growth. Find ways to nurture this inner child and be the parent you wish you had. You can ask it what it needs. An effective way I have found to do this is a writing exercise using your dominant and non-dominant hands. Writing the question to your inner child with your dominant hand and then writing the answer from your inner child with your non-dominant hand helps you to bypass your conscious mind and tap into your sub-conscious. Trust can be built with your inner child by your consistency in contact and your integrity in following through with delivering what it asks of you.*

Part II – The Journey Continues

Total Eclipse of the Heart

11. My Breast Cancer Diagnosis

"And the day came when the risk to remain tight in a bud was more painful than the risk it took to blossom."

Anais Nin

IT WAS SHORTLY AFTER MY 35TH BIRTHDAY in August when I went for my annual physical with my family doctor. She suggested I might want to consider going for something called a 'baseline mammogram'. My mom's breast cancer was diagnosed before she was 50 and before she went into menopause. Apparently those things increased my risk factors. The doctor said normally she would suggest women with a family history of cancer (there were relatives on both sides of my family who died of cancer) go for a mammogram at age 40 instead of the usual 50 recommended by health professionals. Because of my mom's cancer history, the doctor suggested I might want to think about going for a mammogram now. She explained that breast tissue in women my age was very dense and hard to read. By going for one now, they could use it as a normal baseline for comparison when I went again at age 40. She handed me the hospital requisition and said the procedure was optional. I could go now or wait until I was 40. The decision was up to me.

The requisition sat on my counter for several months. With the cancer history in my family I thought there was a good possibility I might get cancer at some point in my life, but I imagined that day would be quite a ways in the future. I did not feel any urgency to go for the mammogram. I was a busy, stay-at-home mom with a five and a two-year-old. There were hardly enough hours in the day as it was. Never mind adding a couple more to go for an examination that ranked right up there as one of women's least favourite health procedures. It just was not a priority to me. To be honest, I did not often put myself on the priority list. Everyone and everything else came first.

Near the middle of December I noticed the requisition again and I decided to book the appointment. I was starting a new year soon and a little voice in my head asked, "Why not begin a new tradition of being proactive about your health?" On January 2nd I went to the hospital and they did a mammogram of both breasts.

Three days later I was going about my normal daily routine. I had just dropped my five-year-old daughter off at kindergarten and put my two-year-old down for a nap when the phone sounded its unwelcome intrusion into my few hours of alone time. The voice on the other end of the line said she was calling from the hospital. They wanted me to come back for another mammogram and an ultrasound. She said the first mammograms they took were not clear enough. In every fibre of my being I knew that 'some point in my life' was now.

Time stopped for me in the surreal way it does in the middle of a life altering crisis. I went into auto pilot as I wrote down the appointment information and hung up the phone. I could barely breathe. I picked up the phone again and tried several times before my hands stopped shaking long enough for me to manage to find the right numbers to call my husband at work. I rarely called him and I was nearly hysterical on the phone. He told me there was no use getting myself all worked up when we did not even know if there was a problem yet. We would just have to wait and see what the results of the second mammogram were. I was stunned. I hung up on him, something I had never done before. Then I called one of my best friends. By that point I was crying so hard I could not speak. She did not need to know why. She just said, "I'll be right over." My husband arrived home about an hour after my girlfriend came over. By then I already made up my mind I could not count on him to help me through this. I would need to make a go of it on my own.

When I got to the hospital for the second mammogram, I registered at the diagnostic imaging department. The clerk at reception wanted to double check with me that the mammogram and ultrasound were for my right breast. The fact they narrowed it down to one breast told me this was more than a routine do over. Once they completed the mammogram, they asked me to wait because the radiologist wanted to talk to me. He told me they found a spot on the mammogram which they were going to also examine by ultrasound, but for me not to worry. The chances of it being breast cancer in a woman my age were very slim. The looks on everyone's faces were telling me a different story. The technician who took me in for the ultrasound looked devastated. I got very familiar with that look. I called it the, 'I am so sorry you are going to die' look.

Now that the tests were done, the wait for the diagnosis began. My test results would be sent to a surgeon. I called my family doctor to see if we could speed up the process somewhat. She reassured me that the likelihood of me having cancer was pretty slim, but she would see what she could do. The woman surgeon she wanted to refer me to was on vacation and would not be back for three weeks. The doctor told me this surgeon would be her first choice. I had the option of going to another surgeon sooner, but something told me to wait.

Much of what happened during the three weeks between mammogram and diagnosis is a blur for me. I died a thousand deaths in my mind and mourned for a life I thought I was not going to have. I worried constantly about what would happen to my children. I played computer games at night after the kids were in bed. Eventually my mind was numb and I would be too exhausted to think about cancer anymore. When I could not keep my eyes open any longer, I would collapse into bed for a few hours of sleep. Each morning as I awoke, the stark prospect of my future would come rushing back to me. I cried in the shower so my daughters would not see me upset all the time.

I was receiving lots of support from friends during that time. Two books found their way into my hands and my heart through these angels. The first was Louise L. Hay's *You Can Heal Your Life*, and the second was Dr. Bernie S. Siegel's *Love, Medicine and Miracles*. Reading Louise Hay's personal story of how she overcame cancer naturally was inspirational. Her book helped me begin to consider how I might have contributed to the development of dis-ease in my body. It gave me hope there were things I could do to help my body heal. Bernie Siegel's book took me on a journey of self-empowerment. His story was a moving account of his work with cancer patients. His respect for the dignity of the person behind the disease really spoke to me. He talked about ECAP groups he facilitated. ECAP was an acronym for Exceptional Cancer Patients. The premise of his book was that attitude had a huge impact on the patient's experience of the disease. Those who believed they were going to die often did. I made a choice to be an exceptional cancer patient! I was going to live each day to the fullest. I might not have any control over the length of time I lived, but I certainly had control over the quality of days I had left. The irony of having to come near to death in order to appreciate life was not lost on me. The truth is none of us know when our number is going to be up. Cancer was a gift in that it was an acute reminder to not take my life or the people in it for granted.

Finally it was time to see the surgeon. My husband came with me to the appointment and coincidentally it was his birthday. I liked the surgeon as soon as I met her, and I was glad I waited. She was straight forward and compassionate. I never felt like I was just a number or a name on a file folder. She encouraged questions and took lots of time to explain things to me. She did a needle biopsy in her office. She said that regardless of whether the results of the biopsy showed the lump was cancerous or not, it was fairly large and she would like to remove it. Then she told me I had a couple of options. If the lump proved to be cancerous I could choose between a mastectomy, or removing only the lump followed by radiation therapy. She said the survival rate for the second option was shown to be comparable to the first. I told her I wanted the breast removed. I did not want to risk the cancer coming back. She said if I were an older woman she would support that option. But, in her opinion, I was still at an age where my breasts were an important part of my identity. If both treatment options were equally as effective her advice would be to keep my breast. I decided to go with her recommendation. She scheduled me for surgery for a lumpectomy and axillary dissection (removing the lymph nodes under the arm closest to the lump) on February 1st. The axillary dissection was to check to see if the cancer had spread to any of the lymph nodes. If it had, then it would have shown the ability to travel and chemotherapy post-surgery would be added to the treatment regimen. She gave me requisitions to take to the hospital for more tests. They wanted to confirm the cancer had not spread to any of my other organs. My husband went with me to the hospital and I had blood work done and a chest x-ray taken. Both were normal. Then we went for a coffee. We sat together as only two people whose entire world has just been turned upside down could. Disbelief hung heavy in the air around and between us. I think he was in his own world of remembering his dad dying of cancer. And I was going down memory lane in my mind of my mother's breast cancer diagnosis and treatment. My husband and I never really talked about anything deep and meaningful before, and this occasion did not suit mundane conversation. I do not think we said very much to each other. I remember thinking that my diagnosis was a terrible birthday present for my husband. We would never forget that date.

The surgery went well. The surgeon held my hand as the anaesthetist was getting ready to put me under. She told me to hang in there and that everything was going to be fine. I thanked her for everything she was doing for me. She told me we were a team, she and I. I liked that thought. It was echoing the message in the books I was reading. I was the co-creator of my experience. When all was said and done the prognosis was not great. The tumour was cancerous. It was large, poorly differentiated, and it had spread to one of my lymph nodes. That meant I was going to have chemotherapy treatments. They were not able to remove a healthy margin of tissue around the tumour because it was right back against my chest wall. The long-term survival statistics were not high and so I asked not to hear them. I had no intention of being a statistic. I could not help but think the little voice inside my head that asked me about being proactive about my health was very wise indeed. If I had waited until I was 40 to go for that mammogram I probably would not have lived.

I came home from the hospital with one breast smaller than the other, stitches, and two drainage tubes: one under my breast and the other under my armpit. The tubes drained into a small bag that needed to be emptied regularly. My mom came down to help look after my daughters while I recovered. She also ended up looking after me. It seemed she and I had come full circle. As a little girl I was the sick child on the couch using the only guise she knew to get her mom to take care of her. Then I was the pissed-off adult/child who purposely refused her care. Now, here I was, an adult allowing her to take care of me. She was a wonderful nurse. She helped me to bathe my wounds and change the dressings and the bag that was collecting the fluid. I took one look at the bruising on my chest and under my arm and I thought I was going to throw up. My mom did not even bat an eye. I did not think about what she must have been going through at the time. Later she told me she was furious with God. Was it not bad enough He had given her breast cancer? But to have visited the same fate on her daughter was almost more than she could bear. I did not know any of that at the time. All I knew was that I was crying out for help, and finally my mother was answering that cry.

My husband was going on a business training course in Atlanta, Georgia for a week in the middle of March. My chemotherapy treatments were not going to begin until March 23rd, so my husband suggested I accompany him to Georgia. He thought it would be a nice break for me before the gruelling treatments began. Our next-door neighbours looked after our girls for us. We had a great time away. We rented a convertible car. It cost more than the regular rentals, but I wanted to be able to feel the wind blowing through my hair before I lost it all with the chemotherapy. He went off to his course each morning, and I went off by myself to explore the city. My usual apprehension in new situations seemed to have disappeared with the cancer diagnosis. I was facing my own mortality. Every other fear I had paled in comparison. I found a t-shirt that said "Attitude is Everything!" Needless to say, I bought it.

I was scheduled for nine chemotherapy treatments spaced three weeks apart, followed by twenty-five daily week-day radiation treatments. The chemotherapy was going to be done first. It was a systemic treatment and was designed to kill any cancer cells that might have travelled elsewhere in my body. They gave me the strongest chemo drugs they had in the highest dosage they could. Because I was young, my cells were multiplying faster: both the good and the bad. The chemo regimen was designed to destroy the bad cells. It also killed the good ones. The treatments were scheduled to start six weeks after surgery. They wanted the incisions from the surgery to heal first.

We had an orientation session at the oncology ward of the hospital. The nurses guaranteed me all of my hair would fall out, and it was likely the chemotherapy treatments would put me into early menopause. They suggested I get my hair cut short and get fitted for a wig. In their experience patients found it easier to do these things before they began to lose their hair. When it began to fall out, shorter hair was not as obvious as it went down the drain in clumps. I got my hair cut and I bought a wig. I thought I was ready. I asked my husband if he was planning to come with me to the treatments. He said, "Of course I am. There's nothing more important than that." I was surprised and also very grateful I would not be doing this part alone after all.

As much as I thought I was ready, I do not think anything can really prepare you for the effects of chemotherapy. I received the drugs intravenously and the treatment took several hours. My husband dropped me at home afterwards. Allison's kindergarten teacher suggested I ask the school district to bus her to school as I would not likely be in any shape to walk her to school during the course of my treatments. After the bus picked her up, I sat down to have an avocado salad for lunch. It was not long before my body began to react to the onslaught of toxic chemicals in my system. As the afternoon wore on my body began to shut down bit by bit. All bodily systems not essential for life support came to a standstill. Digestion stopped, excretion stopped, and I was extremely tired. The nausea was debilitating, but I did not throw up. The food I ate before the treatment stayed in my system. For years afterwards my body associated the taste of foods eaten before a chemo treatment with being sick. I could not eat avocadoes for a long time. I was like the walking dead for almost a week. By the second week my body was beginning to function again. By the third week, just as I was starting to feel a little better, it was time to go for another treatment. I went for blood work before each treatment to determine if my white blood cell count had rebounded enough for my body to withstand another one. There were some weeks when it was touch and go, but I did finish the course of nine treatments. After six treatments I began to throw up. My body had reached its maximum tolerance for the toxins.

In addition to traditional allopathic medicine I sought the advice of a naturopath. I tried all sorts of complementary therapies too: meditation, energy healing, colonics, Essiac tea, and guided visualizations, among other things. I sensed there was more unknown than there was known about cancer. I was going to do everything within my power to stay alive to see my children grow up. I took lots of vitamins and herbs and supplements. Interestingly enough, I did not lose all of my hair or go into early menopause.

I did not have a, "Why me?" attitude about cancer. Mine was more a, "Why not me?" The question I asked myself was, "What am I meant to learn from this disease?" I remember sitting on the porch at the front of my house with a girlfriend who was visiting and saying to her that I did not think I was going to die from breast cancer. She said she had the same feeling.

One of the hardest side effects from the chemotherapy drugs was the hair loss. Even losing some of it was devastating for me. My hair was always a part of my feminine identity. The loss of it became symbolic of all the losses cancer was delivering. I stood crying in the shower one morning and finally surrendered the whole experience. I let go of the illusion of control as I watched pieces of my beautiful hair circle the bathtub drain before they slipped from sight. I talked to God. I stopped asking to beat this thing and instead I began to ask for whatever was best for my children.

My mom and I had a talk about the whole cancer experience. She babysat the girls while my husband and I went to see the surgeon. When we got home I could see she was hoping I would give her good news. When I told her I had breast cancer she said something to me I have never forgotten. She told me that ever since I was a little girl I had never given up on anything. If something stumped me, I was determined, and I kept at it until I figured it out. She told me she was convinced I would beat this thing. Her statement stirred up things inside of me in two ways. Firstly, that she noticed anything about me when I was growing up. I assumed she was too caught up in her own pain to even know I existed. If I was wrong about that, I wondered which of my other judgements about my mother I was wrong about. Secondly, knowing she believed in me really touched my heart.

The challenges of trying to raise two young children while undergoing cancer treatments were many. I hated that I did not have the strength or energy to walk Allison to school. Walking her to the corner and putting my little five-year-old on a big school bus all by herself brought a lump to my throat every time. This was not what I planned. Then to have an active two-year-old at home when some days it was all I could do to get myself out of bed. We watched a lot of children's movies together. I would sit Laken in the reclining chair beside me, and she would watch the movie while I slept. I would wake up if she moved, so I was sure she would not come to any harm.

My husband was the one to suggest we get a cleaning lady while I was undergoing treatments. It was such a treat to come home to a clean house. He also did the grocery shopping. I was very fortunate to have good friends who would drop off pots of soup or offer to take the girls for the afternoon. My girlfriend, who was the one to come over when I got the call from the hospital, had the knack of calling at just the right moment to support me. As much as I had a positive attitude most of the time, cancer was a roller coaster ride for me. There were times when I was at the top of the ride and other times when I plummeted into despair. I was grateful to have found Enya's music. My Celtic heritage spoke to me through her haunting melodies. They reminded me of my connection to my ancestors and the unseen world of Spirit.

There were some friends who disappeared out of my life. It was sometimes surprising for me to see who stuck it out for the long haul, and who could not find it within themselves to stay. I think some people did not call or make contact with me because they did not know what to say. The truth was, what people said really did not matter. What mattered to me was they took the time to connect. I wondered if I reminded some people of their own mortality. Getting breast cancer at 35 was pretty rare then. If it could happen to me perhaps they thought it could happen to anyone.

As much as having breast cancer presented many challenges it also provided many opportunities. It was a complete break from all I knew. Cancer gave me the time to decide what I wanted to add back into my life and what I would let fall away.

Redefining My Priorities

The first order of change was that in fighting for my life, I became a priority on my list of things to do every day. Prior to breast cancer I was not even on the list. I began to look at the ways in which I sold myself again and again in order to be accepted. How many things was I doing in my life in order to please others at the expense of my own needs? My body was telling me in no uncertain terms it had enough. It did so in a way I was sure to pay attention to. I love the story about God trying to get your attention. It begins as a whisper and if you do not pay attention it becomes a tap on the shoulder. If the tap on the shoulder fails, the two by four over the head comes next. The last and most extreme attempt is the house falling down around your ears. Breast cancer was the house falling down around my ears. Now I was listening.

In the months that I was undergoing treatments I did a lot of soul searching. What was my purpose here, and if it turned out I only had a few months to live, what did I want to spend my time doing? The answer was pretty clear for me. I wanted to spend my time with the people I loved. That also meant learning how to love and nurture myself.

Asking for Help

As a child I came to believe the only person I could count on was me. I took that mistaken belief into my adulthood. Breast cancer brought me to my knees and I could not physically do it all myself anymore. It was not so much that I asked for help, as people showered me with it. It was often overwhelming to me emotionally. I was not used to getting that much attention. In so many ways it was impossible to deny, I was being given the message that people cared about me and that I mattered. I was beginning to see the Universe really was a friendly place after all.

I was also learning that accepting people's help was a gift to them, as well as to me. People close to me felt powerless to do anything to stop the cancer. If they could, in some small way, ease my suffering then they felt empowered. I had not really looked at accepting help in those terms before. I thought it meant I was weak, when in actuality it took strength to admit I could not do it all myself. I loved to give to others, but I had not considered that not allowing them to give to me in return created an imbalance in the giving and receiving cycle of life. Even something as simple as receiving a compliment from someone was a challenge before. As I brushed the compliment off, I was blocking the receipt of positive energy. I became aware of this and began to say, "Thank you," instead.

During this time I got a call from a quilting teacher that I had taken a class from when I was pregnant with Laken. She was going to have her work featured in an upcoming quilting book, and she asked if I would consider working with her and making a quilt with one of her patterns. Then my work would also be featured in the book as an example of her student's work. She said it would just be her and me at her house and we could sit out under the tree in her backyard, drink iced tea, and listen to the birds while we quilted. Perhaps the connection to nature and to my creativity would be helpful in my healing process. Although I did not feel well, I also felt a strong pull to create something of beauty amidst the ugliness of cancer treatment. I needed to ask my mom for help babysitting the girls so that I could go. She agreed. It seemed only natural to dedicate the quilt to my mom since I spent many hours stitching on it pondering our relationship.

What Do I Want?

This was a deep question for me and I felt lost in the middle of it. What did I want? I had no idea. I had lots of experiences throughout my life that showed me what I did not want, but almost no idea of what I did want. I spent my whole life up to that point considering the wants of others and arranging my life around them so as to avoid conflict. I was the chameleon in all of my relationships, and I lost sight of me. Breast cancer opened up a window of opportunity to consider this question. I knew for sure I wanted more time, and I wanted to live more authentically in the time I had left. But I did not yet know how to do that or what that would look like.

It Is Okay to Have Feelings and Needs

Feelings seemed as good a place to start as any. In the Adult Children of Alcoholics group, we were offered an exercise to help us identify our feelings. We were given a list of feeling words. We were supposed to stop every hour on the hour during the day and identify what we were feeling at that moment. You may as well have asked me to hang the moon. I knew of four basic feelings: mad, glad, bad, and sad. I had no idea those four consisted of many layers. I buried my feelings from before I was a year old and was using my intellect to keep them buried.

Breast cancer was wearing down all my defences. The chemotherapy drugs were affecting my brain, and my photographic memory appeared to be out of film. Large chunks of my memory were gone, and my ability to use my intellect to shield me from feeling my feelings was impaired. What used to work was not working so well anymore. I had a choice in the middle of this experience to do something different. I began by letting myself cry. I was afraid the tears would not stop. Some days I felt like I was grieving for all the women in my family who were not able to do so. My world did not fall apart as I feared. Instead, each tear helped to cleanse my soul and connect me to those who came before me. Releasing the tears made way for my other feelings to begin to come to the surface. It turned out it was the buried feelings that were keeping me stuck.

As I began acknowledging some of my feelings, my needs began to assert themselves into my consciousness. Along with them they brought old, fearful childhood memories. Trying to get my needs met as a little girl resulted in abuse. It was time to take a new picture here, in more ways than one. First of all, I had to learn it was okay to have needs and to seek to have them met. Then I had to learn to move beyond getting them met in a childlike way. Because I stopped acknowledging my needs around two years of age, my ability to function in this area stayed stuck at a two-year-old level. My expectation was that it was someone else's job to meet my needs. If I wanted to have my needs met in a healthy, mature way, I would first of

107

all have to identify what they were and then find ways of meeting them from the adult part of me.

It was several years later that I discovered David Richo's book, *How to Be an Adult in Relationships*. In it he talked about healthy need fulfillment. My grasp of what he said was that children seek to get their needs met by others 100 percent of the time. Emotionally healthy adults in partner relationships only seek need fulfillment from their partners 25 percent of the time. The other 75 percent of the time they take responsibility for meeting their own needs through varied avenues. This could take the form of themselves, clubs, hobbies, friends, spirituality, and work, to name a few.

It looked like I had my work cut out for me, but at least there was an awareness dawning in me that this area of my life was out of balance.

Identifying My Values

When cancer offered me the perspective of looking at my life as a gift, I started to examine my values. What were they exactly? I adopted my husband's values when I married him because they seemed okay at the time, and subconsciously I wanted to avoid conflict. But abdicating my responsibility for being present in my own life just did not cut it anymore.

I gave a lot of thought to what I was here for and what was significant to me. I tried to make a mental list of what would be important to me at the end of my life. It would make no difference if I had a nice house or a new car. Being buried in designer clothes would not make the life I lived any more meaningful. There was not one material thing I could put on the list. In the final analysis, my relationships with the people I loved were all that mattered. I came to the conclusion I was here to learn how to give love and to receive it. Nothing more, and nothing less.

I even went so far as to consider what I would want the person delivering my eulogy to say. How would they know me for me, or know what to say, if I was a carbon copy or a shadow of someone else's needs, wants, and values. I wanted my eulogy to say I lived a conscious life of compassion, that I loved, and was loved deeply. I wanted it to say it mattered that I was here. I was determined to rediscover the essence of me and then live up to that highest version of my Self.

Finding My Voice

Another part of me that was calling out to be healed was my voice. There were two reasons to stay quiet in my childhood family home. One was that being quiet kept me under the radar and safer around my mother, and the other was that it enabled me to spend quality time alone with my dad. It was like double jeopardy. Not using my voice avoided the bad and delivered the good.

But I was not a child anymore. Whether it was the prospect of a shortened lifespan or nudges from my soul to wake up, I was finding it less and less comfortable to remain silent. If I was not going to speak up for me, who would? I was everyone else's advocate all my life. Now it was time for me to be my own advocate. I started with bringing the word "NO!" back into my vocabulary. Cancer said no for me until I was ready to begin saying it for myself. No one expected someone with cancer to be busy and involved with all the routine activities they participated in before they got sick. As I began to get better, the invitations began to come in again. To be part of this committee, to volunteer at that organisation, to participate in activities my heart just was not into anymore. My first attempts at setting boundaries for myself were messy, just like the 'no' of a two-year-old. With time and practice it became a little more refined. I gave myself permission to respond to invitations with, "I'll need to get back to you about that." This removed the pressure of feeling like I had to make a split-second decision. Then I could take time to consider whether accepting the invitation would bring joy into my life. Time was too short for anything less.

Then I sent a letter to my family doctor. After my breast cancer diagnosis I had not heard a word from her, and I felt like she did not care. I told her I was more than a diagnosis or a patient number on a file. There was a real person attached to those things, and I wanted to remind her of the human side of my experience. To my surprise, she responded very graciously, admitting my diagnosis came as a shock to her, and since she did not know how to deal with it, she had set it aside and not dealt with it. She apologised, and I was very grateful for her acknowledgement of my feelings.

Along with my new found willingness to stand up for myself, I also became acutely aware of sharing good things with people. If I had a message of light or hope, I made a conscious effort to deliver it. Not next week, or next month, or next year, but now. Because there is only now. Tomorrow could be too late.

My Forgiveness Letter to Mom

Between the mammogram and the surgery I had some very prophetic dreams. In one of those dreams my mother died, and I was devastated because I had not told her I forgave her for all the things that happened in our past. The dream felt so real that I awoke in a state of deep grief. As the veil between the world of sleep and wakefulness lifted, I became more grounded in the present moment. I realised it was not too late to offer the gift of forgiveness to my mother and to me.

I wrote the following letter and mailed it to her before my husband and I left for Atlanta. I did not know what my mother would do when she received it. We never talked about her drinking. I was afraid she might never speak to me again, but I hoped it might open up a dialogue between us.

March 8, 1995

Dear Mom,

Just wanted to write to let you know how much I appreciated you coming down to help me after surgery. It's been a long time since I've let you take care of me, and I felt like it was therapeutic for both of us.

I had a dream about you the week after you left. I wanted to tell you about it the second time you came to help, but I never got up the courage to bring up the subject. I thought maybe if I put it in a letter it might be easier for me and I wouldn't forget everything I wanted to say. I thought it might be easier for you too, because it gives you time to deal with what I need to tell you, in your own time and space.

In my dream, you died, and I was devastated. I really regretted that I hadn't taken the time to tell you the things that have been in my heart for the last little while. I took the dream as a sign, that it was time to let you know how I feel. First and foremost, that I love you. I don't know if you know that, in your heart. As all mothers, you are probably riddled with guilt about all the things you wished that you had done differently in the past. I have a lot of those same feelings and I thought now was as good a time as any, to put the past behind us. I wanted to let you know too, that I forgive you for the drinking and the havoc it caused in my life. That's something we never talk about, almost as if we ignore it, it will go away. Unfortunately it doesn't go away, until you deal with it. I've been trying to clear away a lot of the emotional baggage in my life lately, hoping that it will help me to heal, both inside and out. I think the healing in our relationship really began when you stopped drinking with this last bout of cancer. It's an

111

awful disease, but so far I've seen a few positive things come out of it. It's given us a chance to mend some fences, and I don't think there's anything more important than that.

I wanted to let you know that I don't blame you for anything that's happened to me. I realise that you did your best raising me, just as I'm trying to do my best raising my kids, and as I'm sure your mom did her best raising you. When I look back at what little I know about your childhood, and some of the horrors you had to live through, I'm amazed that you survived and have been able to cope as well as you do. It's taken me a long time to realise that your drinking was just a way to try and bury the incredible amount of emotional pain that you must carry around inside of you all the time.

I hope this letter doesn't upset you. This disease has taught me that time is short, and I didn't want either one of us to leave this world behind without forgiving each other for the hurts of the past. I think that will help both of us to heal. I hope we both have lots of time left together to mend some more of those fences. If you'd ever like to talk about any of this; I'm ready when you are! If you'd rather not talk about it, that's okay too, as long as you know how much I care about you.

Love Denise

Mom's Breast Cancer Recurrence

A few days after we returned from Atlanta my mother phoned. All she said was, "I got your letter." I asked her how she felt about it. There were a few seconds where she said nothing. I felt our future hanging precariously in the silence. Finally, she told me there were some things she would talk to me about, but there were some things she would never speak about to anyone. I breathed a sigh of relief that my decision to follow my heart in sending the letter had resulted in the possibility of us forging a different kind of relationship together. I did not want to lose my mother. I told her I would be grateful to listen to whatever she felt she could talk about. When I went to visit her we talked about many things. She said she thought my brothers and I hated her. I told her we did not hate her, I hated how her personality changed when she drank. She told me a little about how she witnessed her father sexually abusing her sisters, and how she always lived in fear of that happening to her. Her father was mean when he drank, and he took out his frustrations on his wife and his daughters. Her mother's only escape from the abuse was illness. She was sick often, and my mother ended up quitting school in grade eight in order to take care of her. We reminisced about how each generation of women in our family did the best they could with the resources available to them, and how each generation had the courage to find progressively more conscious ways to make their lives more bearable. My grandmother used illness to escape an abusive marriage. My mother left my father and her children trying to find herself, in a time in history when she was judged mercilessly for those choices. I sought counselling. We talked about our hopes that my daughters would raise the bar even higher. My mom talked about what it was like to be the youngest of the nine children in her poor farming family. She had a tough life. I was aware that if these were the things she was willing to tell me, the stories she was leaving untold must have been horrendous. She also shared that she never stopped loving my father. I began to have some compassion around how alcohol became a welcome respite from the loneliness, anger, ridicule, and toxic shame she carried inside of her all the time. It was becoming apparent that my mom's abuse of me really had nothing to do with me after all. It was a by-product of her history. Thankfully breast cancer gave us a common bond and a place of vulnerability in which to begin to reconnect.

Not long after we made our first attempt at bridging the gap between us, my mother found out her cancer had metastasised to her liver. I refused to believe she was going to die soon. How could that be possible when I felt like we had just met?

My Mother's Death

Mom began receiving palliative chemotherapy to ease her transition into death at the same time as I was receiving chemotherapy and radiation treatments hoping for a cure. I continued to be in denial. She beat this thing before, surely she could beat it again. Despite my resistance, my mother's health deteriorated rapidly during the last few months of my treatments, and I could not be there for her because it took everything I had to fight for my own life. As my treatments progressed my energy reserves dwindled to almost nothing.

Two days before I finished my radiation treatments my stepfather called in the afternoon to say he had taken my mom to the hospital by ambulance and things did not look good. When I got to the hospital I found out he had not called my brothers, so I did. Mom was still in the emergency room and the on-call physician took me aside in another room. He told me my mom's electrolyte balance was way off and she could go into cardiac arrest. He wanted to know if I wanted them to resuscitate her if her heart stopped. It was at that point I finally understood this was going to be the end of our journey together in this lifetime. I told the physician that I did not know what my mother's wishes were around prolonging life, but she was still coherent and I thought we should ask her what she wanted. She said she did not want her heart restarted.

They finally got her moved to her own room in the palliative care ward. My brothers arrived shortly after that. The nurses began giving my mom heavy doses of morphine for the pain. She drifted in and out of consciousness. I asked the doctor how long he thought my mom would live. He said it was hard to say. She could hang on for as long as two weeks. Armed with that information my brothers and I decided to go home for the night. I knew I needed to get sleep if I was going to be able to be with my mom over the next two weeks. My stepfather said he would stay with her at the hospital. It was important to me she was not alone. I kissed her goodbye and told her I loved her. She said she loved me too, and I headed home.

As I was driving down the highway I began to talk to my father. Even though he had made his transition 18 years before, I had no doubt his spirit was there. I wanted my mom's pain to stop. She still had a lot of anger inside of her, and she was terrified of dying. She was not leaving this world peacefully. I felt like she needed permission to stop fighting and let go. I asked my dad to come and get her and lead her home. I had just climbed into bed when the phone rang. It was my stepfather saying my mom's breathing was not good and I might want to come back to the hospital. When I got there I went into her room. Mom was by herself. I wondered where my stepfather was and then I noticed the machine measuring her vitals was flat-lined. I started to rush out of the room to get a nurse when it finally registered that my mom was dead. Her eyes were still open but all the life was gone from them. I tried to shut them but I could not. Her body felt warm to my touch. I was grateful for that. The last months of her life she said she felt cold all the time. My brothers arrived shortly after I did, and I left them to say goodbye to mom in whatever way felt right to them. We sat at the nurse's station afterward numb with disbelief. We asked what would happen with her body, and they filled us in on the details. I mentioned I had one more radiation treatment to undergo for breast cancer. The nurses could not hold back their tears as they spoke to me. It was like a bad soap opera.

My mom died on a Saturday. On Monday I had my last radiation treatment. It was as if, in her last act as a mother, she willed herself to stay alive long enough to make sure her only daughter was going to be okay. It was not until my brothers and I left the hospital that she allowed herself to let go of her lease on life. She made her transition in time to be an angel on the other side guiding me to wellness after my cancer treatments. My heart was filled with happiness at the thought of my mom and dad's reconciliation. Their love story had a happy ending after all.

Now that the radiation was finished, the real work of figuring out how I was going to live in the world, post cancer, began. While I was undergoing treatments, I was lulled into a false sense of security. I believed the cancer could not possibly come back while I was being treated for it. The scariest part for me happened once the treatments stopped. I said at one point, "Well, it's just you and me now God." In hindsight I see the humour in that statement. In actuality it had been just me and God all along! Not the 'old man with a white beard sitting on his throne in the clouds' God of my childhood, but God in the spiritual sense. This whole journey was about me discovering I was a spiritual being having a human experience, and not the other way around.

There was lots of talk in the cancer world of being a survivor. The consensus seemed to be that if you made it to your five-year checkup without a recurrence, the cancer would be considered to be in remission and you would be called a survivor. My definition of survivor differed from the standard one. I believed whether a woman lived for one month or fifty years after diagnosis, if she lived her remaining days to the fullest then she was a survivor. The 35 years I spent sleepwalking through life prior to my diagnosis could hardly be called surviving. Cancer was my wake up call. I began to survive from the day I was diagnosed. As I continued my healing journey and uncovered more of who I really was, I moved from surviving to thriving.

Sadly, the quilt I dedicated to my mom was not finished before she died. The dedication on the back of it reads, "Your courageous battle with breast cancer taught me much about the strength of the human spirit and the power of love. My soul was with you as I quilted these hearts and flowers and your memory will live on in my heart until we meet again. Love Denise." It hangs in my living room on the wall above my fireplace and is a constant reminder of the possibilities born in love.

Tools for Transformation

- *If you found out you had six months to live, would you change some things in your life? What would you add or let drop away so you could experience more joy? Pick one of those things and begin to work on it.*

- *Are there people in your life you are taking for granted? Find a way to let those people know you appreciate them.*

- *Have you told anyone that you love them today? Have you looked in the mirror and said, "I love you" to yourself today?*

- *Are you on your priority list? What would it take to put yourself on there?*

- *Spend some time considering your wants and needs. Make a list of them and then determine whose responsibility you think it is to meet them. Remember David Richo's premise of 25 percent from a significant other and the other 75 percent from other sources.*

- *Can you identify your feelings? Use the Feelings List in the Resource Section at the end of the book for help.*

- *What are your values? Use the Values List in the Resource Section at the end of the book for help. Can you identify where your values came from? Are they actually yours or have they been handed down by family or society? Have you stopped before to consider their source?*

- *If someone were to write your eulogy, what would you want them to be able to say?*

- *Are you your strongest advocate? When was the last time you said, "No"? Practise in situations that are less threatening and then begin to branch out and set boundaries in other areas of your life. Are there situations where you can compromise with another so both of your needs get met?*

- *Are there people in your life to forgive? Can you write a letter of forgiveness to one of them? It is not necessary to mail it, unless you feel moved to do so. You can also write it and burn or shred it. Just getting it down on paper is often therapeutic.*

Part III – Coming Home

A Shift in Perception

12. Saying Goodbye to the Past

"The real voyage of discovery consists not in seeking new landscapes, but in having new eyes."

Marcel Proust

IN THE MIDST OF ALL THAT WAS GOING ON with my health and my mother's, my husband decided to take a buy-out package from the company he was working for. He sent out many résumés actively searching for another job, but was not having much success. The only company that responded was one in British Columbia. He did not want to move out of the province of Ontario, but he was out of work for several months and had not received any other job offers. We were debating the merits of such a move prior to my mom passing away. Partway through my mom's funeral service I was guided to look up at the wall at the foot of her coffin. Through my tears I noticed an oil painting of mountains hanging there. I took it as a sign from my mom that moving to British Columbia was the next step for me. Mountains were appearing in my life again. They helped me to gain perspective after my dad's death. And now they were calling to me after my mother's passing.

My husband had misgivings about leaving Ontario. We did not know anyone in British Columbia, and most of our family and friends were either in Ontario or Québec. It appeared he was running out of options on the job front though. If we were going to move, our girls were at a good age to do that. Laken was not yet in school and Allison was in grade one. We thought it would be less of an adjustment for them while they were younger. In addition to my brothers, I would be leaving behind my caregivers and the entire support system I had in place for my illness. I experienced both fear and positive thoughts. I did not want to leave my brothers behind, and yet I knew we could still visit. It was not like when we had been in Saudi. I felt guilty that if I moved away I would not be able to pay all the people back who did so many kind things for me when I was sick. Then I began to realise life was not necessarily about paying things back. It could also be about paying them forward. I was sure there would be lots of people in my future I could help in some way. I felt certain the move would be an opportunity to begin a new life with my new perspective on living. I was transforming myself with the changes I was undergoing spiritually after breast cancer. In British Columbia no one would know me. I could be the person I chose to be, with less pressure to conform to expectations of who I used to be. I knew the west coast had a reputation for more advanced thinking in the areas of personal growth. Complementary therapies were more readily accepted and available. I did not know what I might find there, but I knew I had only just begun to uncover my Real Self. I was open to trying new things that would continue to raise my consciousness.

The Move to Langley, British Columbia - Geographical Cure; the Final Frontier

The hiring process with the new company was long and drawn out. My husband went for his first interview in Toronto. He was one of many applicants, and he was short listed from that group. His next interview came a few months later, and this one took place in British Columbia. When they narrowed it down to three candidates for the job and my husband was one of them, the company flew us both out to British Columbia so I could see if it looked like a place I could call home. I welcomed leaving the bleak winter landscape of Ontario behind for a few days. I loved flying over the snow-capped mountains. As the plane descended into Vancouver I could see the ocean. Once I was on the ground, I saw flowers blooming in gardens while I was walking from the airport to the car. The sky was the most intense shade of blue I had ever seen. What was not to like about this place? I felt like I just landed in paradise.

After much discussion about the pros and cons of moving, we decided to pack up our life in Ontario and head west. My husband left ahead of us and began working at the new job in February. I stayed at home in Ontario with the girls so Allison could finish as much of grade one as possible. We joined him in British Columbia on Mother's Day weekend in the middle of May. As the plane was taking off from the runway in Toronto I began to cry. My heart knew I was leaving my hometown, and I would not be back to live there again. The tears were not really sadness. They were more about gratitude for my life up to that point and my deep love for the place where I was born.

The beauty of British Columbia in winter was surpassed by its magnificence in spring. I had never seen so many flowering trees and shrubs. They lined the boulevards and people's beautifully landscaped properties. It seemed like no matter where I was in the greater Vancouver area, mountain vistas would greet me and take my breath away. No wonder they called it 'lotus land'. We travelled to a lot of countries during our time in Saudi Arabia. In comparison, British Columbia was one of the most beautiful places I had ever seen. I could not think of a better place to continue my healing journey.

Personal Growth, Full Speed Ahead

It was not long after our move to Langley that Neale Donald Walsch's *Conversations with God: An Uncommon Dialogue (Book 1)* found its way into my hands. When I read the back jacket of the book, it spoke directly to my soul. Here, finally, was a God of my understanding. There were parts of the book that caused me to weep; such was the feeling of homecoming for me in its pages. It was a personal invitation from Source to enter into relationship. A relationship based on love and equality, not fear and control. Every page was full of opportunities to partner and flow with the Divine by stepping into the Divine part of me, the part that knew no limits.

My appetite for knowledge was insatiable. Now that I was on a path of personal growth, there was no going back for me. As I found new ways of relating that made me feel better, lapses into the old ways of doing things gave me a feeling of deep discord. There were times when I took two steps forward and then a step back. But all in all, as long as I showed even a little willingness to look at things in a new light, windows on new horizons continued to open up. Books almost jumped off of shelves for me. I did not watch television often, but on the odd occasion when I did turn it on, the program would be exactly what I needed at the time. A teacher would appear in my life to illuminate the next piece I needed for my healing. I do not believe anything is random in the Universe. I believe my soul was calling these missing pieces to me so I could fulfill my greater purpose for being here.

After reading the *Conversations with God* series of books, I heard someone quoting a piece of writing done by Marianne Williamson on the Oprah show one day. The words literally stopped me in my tracks with their undeniable truth. It was like she looked inside of me and was illuminating all the dark corners I had not yet found the courage to look at. To my surprise, what I had been hiding in those corners was my magnitude. I always assumed it was my shortcomings.

A theme that kept reappearing with the books I was drawn to was that the material was often based on principles from *A Course in Miracles* (*ACIM*). This profound body of work touches many lives on a very deep level. It is a spiritual book that sets forth text and daily exercises to help you shift your perception from fear to love. It is applicable in all areas of your life. In the introduction it states, "Nothing real can be threatened. Nothing unreal exists. Herein lies the peace of God." Although Christian based, it deals with universally applicable spiritual themes. I was drawn to it and sought out a copy. When I first opened it and began to read, I was challenged somewhat by its language. It was difficult to read, in a similar way Shakespearean English is. God was referred to in the masculine which I did not believe was true. My childhood experience with Christian-based religions was that they were patriarchal, exclusive, and fear driven. I developed an aversion to Christianity. Or perhaps it would be truer to say my aversion was more about how some people practised exclusivity and called it Christianity. That was not a concept of God I could relate to. I believed in spiritual inclusion, of all races and all religions. I set the book aside on my bookshelf. It was obviously not time for me to read it yet. It would be another four years before I could set aside my judgements and open myself up fully to its messages.

I was really enjoying the tremendous amount of learning I was doing. Even in the midst of the enjoyment, I went through periods of anxiety and unrest. At times I did not want to start anything new that required a long term commitment because I did not know how much time I had left. And at other times I pushed myself relentlessly because of the time factor. I knew there was a reason why I was still alive. I feared that if I did not discover what my purpose was soon, time would run out before I could fulfill it. I shifted back and forth on this 'time' merry-go-round often. I had not yet discovered there really was nowhere I needed to get to. There was only the here and now, and I was already there. Fully inhabiting where I was in the moment needed to happen before the external manifestation of my Divinely guided purpose could unfold.

Tools for Transformation

- *Have you noticed the signs you receive in your life to let you know you are either on the right track, or you have gotten lost along the way? What form do those signs take for you? According to the study of neuro-linguistic programming (NLP) there are three learning styles, or ways we take in information. We are primarily either visual (see messages), kinaesthetic (feel messages), or auditory (hear messages). See if you can discover which learning style is dominant for you.*

- *When you receive a kindness from someone have you ever thought of paying it forward to someone else? Take a moment this week and do something kind for someone. It can even be anonymous if you choose. Watch how brightening up another's life also brightens up yours.*

- *What books and other resources have really helped you? List some of the teachers who have come into your life. Remember that the people who have upset you the most are your greatest teachers. They are showing you the places in you that need healing. When have you been a teacher through your own struggle? There is a list of resources at the end of the book that have been guides on my journey.*

- *How would you describe your experience of time? Can you be in the here and now for very long? Or does your mind take over fairly quickly and deliver you to worrying about the past or anticipating the future? See if you can spend 1 minute (yes…60 whole seconds!) each day this week totally focused on the present moment. Each time your mind wanders in that minute, gently take it by the hand and bring it back to the now.*

13. Travelling to the Core of Innocence in Me

"The holiest of all the spots on earth is where
an ancient hatred has become a present love."

A Course in Miracles

AS I SETTLED INTO MY NEW LIFE in British Columbia, I began to heal at many levels. My body was slowly beginning to repair itself. My spirit felt at home amongst the giant cedar and fir trees, and the ocean seemed to call my name. My mind, however, was still caught up in the whole concept of time being finite, and of my not having enough of it. I felt frozen in place, not necessarily going backward, but not moving forward either. I heard of a counsellor who dealt specifically with breast cancer patients, and I called her. She worked from a mind/body perspective which fit in with some of my new philosophies. I was discovering how incredibly powerful my mind was, and how it affected my body. I wanted to use my mind to create the life of my dreams instead of staying stuck in the past.

With the counsellor I received validation for the incredible journey I was on up to that point. She listened to my fears for the future, and she did not discount them. I felt heard there. She also did not support the fears, but instead helped me reframe them in order to see the possibilities. I believed I survived cancer for a reason, and I was afraid I would not figure out what that reason was before my time ran out. I felt like I needed to be doing something big with my life in order to honour the gift of my life. The counsellor helped me to reframe the 'something big' and see how working towards my goal of learning how to give and receive love was big. There really was nothing more important in life and there was no set timeframe for it. Reframing the fear lessened its power and helped me to get on with my life.

One of the many things she said, that has stayed with me, was that she believed people do not change. That stopped me dead in my tracks. My whole game plan was about changing my behaviours that no longer served me. What did she mean by saying people do not change? She must have read the look of disbelief on my face and known she hit a nerve. She went on to explain that her belief was people do not change who they are fundamentally. We are all born innocent and then life happens. Finding peace is not about trying to change what is innate. It is about learning to accept all of our idiosyncrasies while finding our way back to that innocent core of who we are. It is a process of shedding the layers we have accumulated that no longer reflect the truth of who we are. Behaviours can be changed but the core of us cannot. What she said affected me deeply. I was not broken, and I was not alone in this process. I had collected baggage from my past, but I could set it down if I chose to. This felt more doable than trying to change who I was. Travelling to the core of the innocence in me was the real journey home.

Unease about my marriage began to come to light in the counselling sessions. It was not a relationship that was emotionally healthy, and my partner was not joining me in my spiritual growth journey. I was getting the first warning bells in my head that the marriage might not be forever. I shut that intuitive voice down quickly. That was not a place I was prepared to go at that time. I was still recovering from breast cancer, and I did not have the physical or emotional strength to even consider being a single mother. I wanted my kids to live in a two-parent home. When I got married, I intended to live happily ever after with this man. I was not yet ready to let go of that dream. I would find a way to make it work, at all costs.

The counselling helped me to ground myself in my strengths. I started to think about the Adult Children of Alcoholics group counsellor asking me if I ever considered being a counsellor. When I looked back at my life, I thought about how many times complete strangers came up to me and told me their life story. I received so much from so many people over the last several years, and I wanted to be able to give back in some way. Counselling seemed like it might be a logical way to do that. I registered for the first class in a Counselling Support Skills program at a local university college. If I was able to complete the classes required, I would be qualified to counsel in two years.

I loved learning, and the classes were teaching me so much. What I had not counted on was that the subject matter of the classes would bring up more of my unresolved issues. As I was learning about what healthy psychological functioning looked like, I was comparing my own life to the norms. I could see where I had progressed in many areas, and I could also see where some of the stumbling blocks were in my quest for a happier life. Again, my marriage was coming to the forefront as one of those blocks.

When I was in high school, I dreamed of post-secondary education but knew my family did not have the funds to make that possible, so I let that dream go. To my delight, I did end up finishing the Counselling Support Skills program and felt a great sense of accomplishment. Not only had I lived a childhood dream, but I was the one who made it possible for myself as an adult. Perhaps it was never too late to grow up. As I was following more of my dreams and bringing more of the real me to everything I did, time became less of an issue for me. Each year that passed with a clear check-up at the cancer centre bolstered my hopes that there would be yet another year to discover more of the authentic me.

I decided I did not really want to work for someone else. When I investigated the possibility of opening my own counselling practice it appeared I would need a Master's degree in psychology. I looked into programs to further my education. All of them included some classes that I was not interested in taking and that had nothing to do with psychology. Or the programs were located in another country. Then I found a local program that taught transpersonal counselling psychology over three years with the option to add further study for a Bachelor of

Arts (BA) undergraduate degree. All the classes related to counselling, and I could be part way to my Master's degree when I finished. Three years sounded like a long time, but I knew if I did not take the program, there was a possibility I would live another three years and then kick myself because I had not signed up. In other words, the three years were going to go by whether I did the program or not. Why not spend the three years moving towards another one of my dreams. I loved that the program description spoke my language of personal growth. It took things to a transpersonal level. That is what I believed my cancer experience helped me do. Go beyond the limits of the ego and the personality for a bigger perspective on life and my place in the world. When I looked at the book list for the courses, I realised I either had most of the books in my personal library, or I had already read them. This program seemed to encapsulate everything I searched out on my own during my healing journey. I signed up for the three years.

The foundation of the transpersonal part of the curriculum was from *A Course in Miracles* (*ACIM*). Now would be the time for me to take my *ACIM* book off my bookshelf, dust it off, and begin to read it. A lot of the counselling part of the program was based on Dr. Murray Bowen's family systems theory of therapy. I read about this briefly in a *Theories of Counselling* class in the two-year counselling program I took, but we had not studied it in any depth. The premise of Bowen's theory is that the family is an emotional unit, meaning that everything that goes on in a family is driven by the emotions of, and the relationships between, all of the members in that family. He believed an individual can be best understood in the context of their place in their family system. Things such as their birth order and what roles they play to help the family function, need to be considered, because each person does not operate in their life alone. Each member of the family is connected, somewhat like a mobile you hang over a baby's crib. When one thing changes on the mobile, the rest of the mobile shifts to bring itself back into balance. At least a three-generation perspective is necessary to view predictable patterns of interpersonal relationships that connect the functioning, or dysfunctioning, of the family. It made sense to me to study people from a systems perspective. After all, the world appeared to operate in systems, from simple cells to more complex forms such as organisms and societies. Each part in the system had its individual role. If you wanted to better understand that role, you really could not view it in isolation. To get a bigger picture and to understand behaviour you needed to view the whole system in operation. Each part contributed to and affected the whole. The beauty of Bowen's theory is that as one individual in a family begins to improve their personal level of functioning it impacts the whole family in a positive way.

Families are complex social systems. The interdependence between the individuals that make up the whole family enable it to function or to dysfunction, as was the case in my family. Each person in my family was connected and joined together in a web of relationships. In order for me to better comprehend my family system, I would need to look at the individual parts we played and also look at my family as a whole. How did all of the parts come together in my family? What were our patterns of interacting? I was beginning to understand why my distancing did not work. Geographical cures and cut-off did not change my partners or my steps in my family dance. All they did was change my physical location. I could not operate outside of my family system, because I carried it with me all the time. Change would only result from my relating differently within the system.

Another interesting aspect of systems is that they are dynamic and tend toward homeostasis. This means the survival of the whole depends on the system maintaining equilibrium and balance. Within families there are often energetic imbalances that have been crying out to be healed for years. Unresolved emotional issues keep appearing in generation after generation until they are resolved. If one member of the family begins to change their behaviours all the other members of the family are affected. I began to get curious about where I fit into my family system and what unresolved emotional issues came down through the generations to land on my shoulders to be resolved.

Bowen also stressed something called differentiation of self. This entailed a psychological separation of heart and mind. Differentiated people can recognise their feelings and be objective observers, choosing whether or not to act on them. Levels of differentiation are determined by the individual's autonomy of self from others. Can they stand for what they believe in no matter how other family members feel? How much can they respond rather than react in stressful situations when anxiety in the system is high? Examining and resolving conflicts at an individual and family level became a lifelong learning process for me.

This counselling program stressed that effective counsellors could not take clients anywhere they had not gone themselves emotionally. We began to unravel our own family systems and we did lots of experiential processes to uproot our unresolved emotional issues. The next steps in my healing journey were the experiential component of healing, exploring my own family history, and moving the trauma out of my body.

Cleaning Out the Cobwebs and Finding My Family

Researching my genealogy was one of the defining moments of the program for me. I did not have much family history and both of my parents were no longer around to answer questions. I decided to try looking up my mom's maiden name in genealogy sites on the internet. I was shocked to discover that my extended family's history was recorded back to 1786. Because I cut off from them when I was 13, their existence was of no consequence in my mind. What I knew of the incest, alcoholism, and abuse in my grandfather's generation disgusted me. I had not even considered there might have been generations that came before them. The computer screen in front of me was telling me something different.

My abusive grandfather and his brother, who sexually abused several girls in the family, were somebody's sons! They were babies once. They were not born incestuous, addicted, and abusive. What had happened in previous generations, that was being reenacted in this one? Finding that they had a rich history began to shift my perception somewhat. They immigrated to Canada in 1856 to become pioneers on land in a little town in Ontario. My great-grandfather was born in 1869. Three years later his mother and his grandmother died within a day of each other. I do not know if it was illness or accident. What is apparent from the records is that at three years of age my great-grandfather lost both his mother and grandmother. I can only imagine how difficult life must have been for pioneering families. Clearing land and living at the mercy of nature. What would happen to a little boy without the protective arms of the most important women in his life? Were the emotions of those great losses ever spoken about or dealt with? I suspected not, as I did not know any of this history. It was as if both the emotions and the losses were buried with these women. I wondered what happened to that little boy and his siblings once their mother died. I felt some empathy for them. The history showed that at some point the family relocated some 200 kilometres away. What would cause a family to leave land they cleared, with their blood, sweat, and tears, and move to another parcel of land they would again have to clear? I did not have answers, but I had lots of questions.

I found the courage to begin to ask the questions of my brothers and any members of my extended family that I could find. I wanted to understand what we were carrying energetically. The pieces came to me little by little as I was ready to process them. I learned that both my mother and my father were unwanted children. My dad's mother tried to abort him at the beginning of her pregnancy, and my mom was always told she was a mistake. Her mom was 50 and starting into menopause when she discovered she was pregnant with her. She thought she was not able to have any more children. There were only two 'good' men in the family system, and they had cut off from the family. The rest abused either themselves or others. The good ones gave up and/or checked out physically or emotionally. I was searching for my own 'good' man to make up for that. Talk about putting pressure on my husband! The only people I knew of in my family at that time who went for post-secondary education, were my stepgrandfather and me. Most of the others did not finish high school. My grandmother on my mom's side used to 'get sick' when it was time for her husband to come home from logging camp. He would then turn to his daughters to satisfy his sexual needs. Her relationship with her daughters was one of subconsciously sacrificing them, and my mother left me unprotected with the same uncle who tried to rape her. The subliminal message from both sides of my family was to give up before I started because anything good was only going to be taken away from me anyway. The pattern on both sides was to sacrifice either Self or other for the family system, either figuratively or literally (suicide, breast cancer, sexual abuse). Women did not have a voice. They kept the family secrets.

What did all of this leave me with? I carried the mantle of making up for the losses on both sides of the family. I was the 'wanted' child, the saviour, the one who was going to make up for all of the lost dreams that had gone before. I was the 'smart' one. The one who was going to get an education and prove my parents were okay. I was going to find the one 'good' man no one else had yet been able to find, while at the same time receiving the message that men are either not there when you need them, or they abuse you. And I was trying to make up for the loss of not being a good enough mother.

All of this gave me a greater understanding of the crushing energetic weight I often felt on me. It also gave me hope, because the dawning of this new understanding presented the possibility of shifting these emotional patterns. This was quite a departure from my state of mind prior to doing the research. Although I did not know it at the time, the part of my heart I hardened against half of my heritage, was beginning to soften a little. I did not have to agree with their behaviour for a spark of compassion to be ignited in me and for the door to forgiveness to begin to open.

Tools for Transformation

- *What is your relationship to time? Do you believe there is lots of it, or not enough? How does that affect how you live your day to day life?*

- *Have you ever considered that what is at your core is innocence? I guarantee you that it is. If you are having trouble seeing it, find a picture of yourself as a baby. Look into that baby's eyes and see if you can find that innocence there. Keep that baby picture where you can see it.*

- *Are there any areas of your life that your intuition is asking you to change?*

- *What are your strengths? Make a list of at least 10 and keep the list on your refrigerator. Any time you begin to doubt yourself, review the list.*

- *Do you have a buried childhood dream you could resurrect now that you are an adult? What step could you take towards making that dream a reality? Can you make a choice that your dreams and goals are more important than the fear?*

- *Are you aware of unresolved emotional issues in your family of origin? What might they be? Is there something you can do in your own life to begin to address how this impacts you?*

- *Are there areas of your life where a shift in perception might ignite a spark of compassion or open a door to forgiveness? List one area and see if you can trace it back emotionally in your family system.*

14. Moving From Fear to Love

"Thoughts rooted in fear will produce one kind of manifestation on the physical plane. Thoughts rooted in love will produce another."

Neale Donald Walsch

ONE OF THE MOST IMPORTANT LESSONS I learned from *A Course in Miracles* (*ACIM*) was that love is our natural state of being. In every moment we are either in a state of love or in a state of fear. There is no middle ground. It is either one or the other and it is not possible to be in both at the same time. Our behaviour is a reflection of which state we are in. If we are coming from a state of love our behaviour is an expression of love and compassion. If we are in a state of fear our behaviour becomes a cry for love. In our human systems we are longing to return to our natural state of love. In the first 35 years of my life I inhabited a place of fear, and my behaviours were a cry for love. It was a space of darkness and belief in lack, where I forgot the truly amazing being I was. After breast cancer I began to open up my eyes and my heart with a willingness to consider a different way of life. Love was where I wanted to live. The more willing I was to see something different, the more new possibilities came into my life. With each one I got to choose who I wanted to be. I got to choose the behaviour that would help me to express the light at the centre of who I am.

Fear - My Old Friend; Changing Our Relationship to Fear

There are some feelings of fear that serve us. The gut feeling that a person, place, or thing is not in our best interest. Then there is the abstract fear that comes from a place of defence inside of us, a type of pervasive anxiety that hangs over us like a dark cloud. I still visit this kind of fear sometimes, but it is not a place where I want to set up house.

Two letters to fear:

June 12, 2000

I could write a book about fear. I've spent close to 40 years wallowing in it. Up until a few years ago it was the guiding force in my life. A life lived in pain and perceived lack.

I'm beginning to understand much more clearly where the perception of lack comes from. The feeling of never being good enough. Not good enough to keep my father from committing suicide, not good enough to keep my mother from drinking, not good enough to make my husband get some of the big truths in life.

A childish perspective, no doubt, but one that served me well as a child. A method of self-preservation.

The fear of abandonment. That I am not good enough to stick around for. Made for a really lonely isolated childhood. But it no longer serves me if becoming an authentically powered human being is who I want to become.

Quite a course I've set for myself. To choose love instead of fear. To choose joy instead of pain. To let go of perceived risk, and trust. Trust that where I am now is exactly where I'm supposed to be on my path. To believe that I am worthy, I deserve abundance and love and that the Universe will provide.

I am so thankful for all the life lessons I've learned so far and I look forward to the challenge of all the new lessons I have yet to master.

March 27, 2010

Hello fear, my old friend. I know I don't often refer to you as "friend", but I'm wondering if we can redefine our relationship. We've been together for so long, you and I. From before my birth, actually. And in all the times we've danced together I haven't ever really thought of you as a partner...but more as an adversary. A foe to be vanquished, a dirty little secret to be hidden away...especially in front of others, garbage to be tossed out or burned or buried. And yet, no matter how much I attempt to slip out of your grasp, you remain in the shadows, waiting for me always.

If I were to put on a different pair of glasses when we meet, would my perception of you change? Could we become acquaintances first? Could we look each other in the eye, however briefly? If I stopped fighting you would you open up and show me your gifts? Could we learn a new dance, you and I? I'm ready to enter into a more loving relationship together.

The first letter about fear was impersonal and did not really address the fear head on. It was more like I was skirting around the edges of the issue and looking for a safe entry point in. This was how I lived my life then. The second letter was much more direct, up close, and personal. The change in my approach made a world of difference in my ability to get to the heart of the matter. It was in redefining my relationship to fear that I began to shift it. Fear and I have danced together in many lifetimes and will dance together in many more. If I stop the struggle and surrender, I can look at fear as a messenger and not as truth. Then the power of choice as to what to do with its messages remains with me.

When I looked at the behaviours that were not serving me, they were inevitably coming from a place of fear. Fear of lack; fear of not being good enough; fear of rejection. The list could go on and on. The clear indicator that I was coming from a place of fear was when I was in reaction to someone or something. Whenever I had the proverbial finger pointed in blame, certain I was justified in my anger, it became a flag for me that something from my past was being triggered. This was truly a gift because the first step in shifting from a state of fear to a state of love was the awareness I was in fear. Fear actually served as my awareness barometer. Once I could identify a trigger, it was up to me to explore what the trigger was, and to do my work to get to the bottom of it. It was an opportunity to dig a little deeper into myself. Each time I would discover, that how I felt, really had nothing to do with anyone, or anything else. As soon as I made someone or something outside of me responsible for my happiness, or lack of it, I gave my power away and ended up feeling like a victim. I discovered I was powerful, and I could choose to use that power from a place of love or a place of fear.

Returning to Love

Those three words soothe my soul. They speak of homecoming to me. I feel comforted there. I feel held there. I feel at one there. In that place of love I know all things are possible. There is no us and them. There is no better than or less than. There is only inclusion, acceptance, connection, and oneness with All That Is.

I am not talking about romantic partner love here, but something so much bigger than that. I am talking about pure joy, an internal state of being at peace with yourself, the world, and your place in it. A state of recognizing the spark of Divinity within you and acting from that state in all you do. There is no external substitute for this. Sometimes we try to recreate it through amassing material possessions, through addictions, or through romantic partner relationships. But none of those things can be substitutes for the real thing. We may get a temporary high from them, but it does not last. Once it wears off we are on to the next person or thing we think is going to do it for us. What I discovered through my search is; what I was looking for was inside of me all along.

I used to think this state of being was reserved for gurus, or masters, or at the very least someone who meditated on a mountain top for several years. It has come as a great surprise to me to learn that love is always a choice in every moment, for everyone. And when we realise we have missed the mark and have dropped back into that state of fear, we can choose to stay there for a while, or we can make another choice. We can ask ourselves, "What would love do here?" Then take our next step from that place. I am not saying it is always easy, because there are times when it takes everything I have to make another choice. My ego often wants to be right, no matter what. As long as I am convinced I am right, I have closed myself off to the possibility of continued learning. If I can sit in a place of not knowing, I can be open to what the Universe is trying to show me. It is often really uncomfortable for me to be there. When I drop into some of those deep places of fear that I have known since I was a child, it can feel like I have no other choice but fear. I feel vulnerable there and my natural inclination may be to defend against that vulnerability. I considered vulnerability a weakness when I was a child. I see now it takes courage to choose to stand in that vulnerable place, naked before the world. We are most alike in our vulnerability. That is the universal soft spot in us from which true connection is possible.

There is always a choice in how we interact in the world. And we are humans who are works in progress. I am learning to be patient with myself and remember we are all entitled to the time it takes to learn.

Moving from Head to Heart

My head was my refuge from my heart for many years. As long as I stayed tangled up in my intellect I could avoid moving into the feelings I was afraid would swallow me alive. I could analyse a problem to death for days, or months, or years on end and never really touch on the deeper meaning of it. Nor would the analysing do anything to solve the problem. I literally made a career of analysis. Many times I was brought into a company to organise their administration departments so things ran smoothly. One of my first jobs was as an inventory controller. Control was my leftover game from childhood. If I could control it, whatever *it* was, then my belief was there would not be any surprises.

I have heard it said the longest journey we will make is the one from our head to our heart. In my case that is literally about 38 centimetres. But when I began this emotional journey it felt like 38 kilometres. And I was not running to get there. I was taking baby steps, sometimes crawling when the going got tough. The catalyst for the pilgrimage to the centre of my being was my dark night of the soul. Losing my mind was the first step to finding my heart! There was nowhere else to go but my heart. In that place, I experienced that control was an illusion at best. There was a grander plan for me than I could have dreamed of, if I was willing to let go of the small plans I was holding onto.

Integrating Head and Heart - How to Use Our Heads While Following Our Hearts

As in all things in life, balance is the key. To me the mind and the heart are polarities on the same spectrum. The analytical driving mind is a function of the left side of our brain, and our compassionate receptive heart is governed by the right side. If we function solely in one or the other our life becomes one dimensional and lacking in depth and perspective.

Finding the balance between the two was much like the polarity swings I went through to come to a place of 'good enough mothering'. As a child I learned to survive by living strictly in my head which kept me in fear and away from the richness and vibrancy of life. Once I rediscovered my heart as an adult, the pendulum swung way over to the other side of the spectrum, and I was a bucket of mush. I loved everyone and wanted to save the world. I would give my time and energy to others indiscriminately which would lead to me burning out. Then I would withdraw to my head to regroup. Over time as I learned to take better care of myself, the swings between the two became less pronounced and I found my place somewhere in the middle.

I have discovered one of the things that keeps me stuck in my head is asking the question, "Why?" While there is value in understanding something, staying stuck in the 'why' can result in my authoring all sorts of stories in my mind that may or may not have any resemblance to reality. 'Why' allows me to circle around in my head questioning the natural order of things. It really does not matter why something has happened. All that matters is what is, and dealing with that in the present moment. More effective questions would be, "How do I feel about this and what can I do to bring more love into this situation?" In that way I am proactively accessing my heart through my feelings, and I am using my head to determine the course of action that will bring more light into the world.

Expansion Rather Than Contraction of the Heart

Asking the 'how' and 'what' questions expand my heart in love rather than contracting it in fear. It is in the expansion that I can reach and teach others. It is in this place I find joy, because it is here that I am extending joy to others. *ACIM* teaches that the only thing missing in any situation is what we are not giving to it.

As I gained more experience in balancing my head and my heart, it became easier for me to open my heart and trust that everything that came into my life was in some way for my highest good. Nothing was being done to me; rather, circumstances for growth were being offered to me. The trust was not dependent on the actions of others. The ultimate trust was about me and recognizing I had the resources within me to handle whatever life might dish up.

In all situations I had the option of expanding my heart in love or contracting it in fear. The choice was mine regardless of what was going on around me. I found it is possible to stand calm and solid in the centre of my world while life storms all around me. Not only is it possible, it is necessary if I want to experience lasting peace. Standing calmly and solidly requires that I know the Truth of who I am and what I stand for. It requires a remembrance that I am not alone on this journey. Using the tools for transformation in each of the chapters leading up to this point, together with the information in Chapter 22, will give you more clarity around this.

An expanded heart is a soft place. It is a welcoming, open energy. There is an opportunity to connect with others and your higher Self in that place. By contrast, a contracted heart gives the clear message of "do not enter". The channels of giving and receiving are pinched off and life force energy gets blocked. In the Eastern naturopathic traditions there are seven major chakras (energy centres) in the body that are located from the crown of the head to the tip of the tail bone. The heart chakra is in the middle, with three chakras above it and three chakras below it. The heart chakra is often considered the centre of the human energy system, where the energy of the Divine meets the human part of us. Keeping the heart expanded and open allows us to access the Divinity within us and receive higher wisdom, and it gives us a grounded place from which to nurture ourselves and others.

Focusing on the Light and Allowing
the Darkness to Recede on Its Own

Most of my years in this lifetime I have chosen to valiantly battle the darkness, doing everything within my power to keep it at bay. Much like my old dance with fear, all of my energy was drained away in the battle. There was not much energy left for anything else. That same pattern went on in my family for generations, until I was introduced to the concept of focusing on the light and allowing the darkness to recede on its own. In essence, Spirit asked me to lay down my sword and consider the possibility there might be another way to go through life. As much as my ego was terrified of the idea, my soul sighed with knowingness and relief. I could choose to focus my energy on the light that had always been there. I had not seen it because I was too busy battling the dark. I thought of the way a lit candle illuminates an aura all around itself. The candle is not expending any effort to dispel the darkness. It shines what it is, and by virtue of it being itself, what surrounds it is changed.

I could choose to perceive that the world was full of darkness or I could change my perception. I could let go of the illusion and focus on what was real. This did not mean denying there were dark things happening in the world. It meant there was also much that was good. As I put my attention and my energy into those things that were filled with light, my world began to reflect that back to me and I began to manifest more light into my life.

Tools for Transformation

- *Take some time over the next week and see if you can become aware when your behaviour is coming from a place of love and when it is coming from a place of fear.*

- *What is your relationship to fear? If you would like it to change, consider writing a letter to it expressing how you feel.*

- *Do you have a finger pointed in blame anywhere in your life? Can you identify what the trigger is for you in that situation? Can you trace the trigger back to an earlier time in your life? What might need to be healed there?*

- *Are there external sources you are using as a substitute for accessing the spark of Divinity within you?*

- *Is there a person, place, or thing in your life right now that could use an infusion of love? What step could you take to make that happen?*

- *Have you ever allowed yourself to be vulnerable with another? What feelings come up inside of you in that place? Can you sit with the feelings long enough to allow them to dissipate on their own?*

- *Are you predominantly a heart dweller or a head dweller? What can you do to create more balance in this area?*

- *Take some time to notice if your heart is in an expanded or contracted state most of the time. If it is contracted, see if you can sit quietly for five minutes a day and send loving energy to your heart.*

- *Are you weary from battling the darkness? In small increments can you begin to lay down your sword and focus your energy on something of light in your life?*

15. Separation and Divorce

"Do the thing you fear the most and the death of fear is certain."

Mark Twain

AS I CONTINUED IN MY PERSONAL GROWTH work, the relationship between my husband and I slowly unravelled. I assumed because he witnessed my transformational journey through cancer, he also accompanied me on the emotional part of it. Time revealed to both of us that was not the case. He watched me grow in leaps and bounds and said he felt admiration to be witnessing my process. But he very honestly revealed to me that he did not think he could come with me.

My soul searching after cancer led me to make a lot of shifts in my life. Once I began to put myself on the priority list, my behaviours began to change. I was settling for the status quo and that just did not cut it anymore. So here we were in our 18th year of marriage, and the woman my husband thought he partnered with for life was gone. In her place he had the 'real' me. That was not what he signed on for when he said, "I do." Once I unearthed my values, I could not go back to the way I was living my life before cancer.

A large part of our marriage was based on acquiring material goods, as if that was somehow a measure of success. I had a different measure of success now. My goal was to learn how to give love and receive it. As long as I was taking steps towards that goal I felt successful. Much like my idea of what constituted a cancer survivor; not how long we lived after diagnosis, but that we lived each day to the fullest. More was not necessarily better. My husband told me he felt like he was a failure. He was not where he anticipated he should be by that point in his life. We were both driving cars that were several years old, and our house was not as large or as new as he would have liked. I told him I was grateful to even have a vehicle, and I would live in a tent on a beach with him. The material stuff just did not matter to me anymore. But it still mattered to him. I used to preface my attempts at changing his way of thinking with the expression, "In the grand scheme of things..." That drove him crazy.

This was just one of many fissures that were appearing in the carefully glossed exterior we presented to the world. Another was that he was the quintessential dreamer and I was the quintessential pragmatist. It felt to me like he had his head in the clouds, and it probably felt to him like I was an anchor around his feet. He was the extravert, and I was the introvert. He wanted to try new things, and I preferred the tried and true. All of the things that attracted us to each other in the beginning of our relationship now appeared to be driving us apart. Money was a constant source of conflict. Our bank account went into overdraft every month. My perception was that he spent money on things we did not need, and his perception of me was the same. Each of us was sure we were right. That need to be right was coming from a lack of confidence and a lack of authentic power in both of us. If we truly believed in ourselves we would not have felt the need to try to change each other's mind.

It felt like the more I tried to step into the new me, the stronger my husband's attempts became to try to keep things the way they were. We were both angry. I kept my anger inside and it leaked out in passive-aggressive ways. He expressed his outwardly and loudly. This felt too similar to the anger in my family of origin, and I would immediately shut down, anticipating danger. At one point in an argument he shouted, "Who are you?" He felt like I turned into someone he did not know. To be fair to him, I had. When we met and married I was wearing many masks. I turned myself into whoever he wanted me to be. I was in the process of removing the masks and the layers I accumulated throughout my life. Underneath them the authentic me was finding her way to the surface more and more.

My tolerance for the continued use, and sometimes abuse, of alcohol in our home decreased substantially. I felt like I had subconsciously recreated walking on eggshells, exactly like what I had experienced in the chaotic environment of my childhood home. I sought out and began to go to Al-Anon meetings. These meetings are a fellowship of Alcoholics Anonymous geared towards the families of alcoholics. I found a meeting specifically for Adult Children of Alcoholics. There I learned I could not change anyone's behaviour but my own. I realised I had been engaged in a co-dependent alliance with my husband for years. I allowed my well-being to be dependent on his being happy. I sacrificed my needs to make that happen. It was time for me to start taking accountability for my own happiness. It was time for me to grow up.

I was still seeing the counsellor. She suggested a couple's workshop that would help us deal with the conflict in our relationship. It took me several weeks to work up the courage to ask my husband to go to it with me. We had not done any personal growth work together in that format. I knew I would be asking him to step way outside of his comfort zone. I also knew if we did not do something, our marriage would be over. I finally told him I felt like we were drifting farther and farther apart and I did not know how to change that. I suggested the workshop and, to his credit, he agreed to go.

In the workshop we looked at many things. One exercise involved us drawing up a conflict agreement together. In another exercise we looked at our values. This was most revealing. When we listed our values in the order of their priority, what was on the top of my list was on the bottom of his list, if it was on his list at all, and vice versa. We had a few common values in the middle, family being one of them, but in general we were miles apart.

The workshop did not make any promises of keeping us together. Though it did give us tools to negotiate conflict. If it ended up that we separated we could do that in a more civilised manner if we chose to. Part of the workshop was a one-hour couple's counselling session with the therapist who led the workshop. When she talked to me she asked about my cancer experience. She said it was fairly common for cancer patients to begin to distance emotionally from the people they loved, so it would not be so hard for their loved ones when they died. She asked me if that was my experience. It was the first time I thought about it, but that had indeed occurred for me. She asked me if I had come back yet, and my honest answer was, "No." So, as much as I was blaming my husband for distancing from me with anger and alcohol, I was an equal partner in the distance dance by withdrawing emotionally from the relationship.

The fact he even agreed to come to the workshop was exciting for me. When we came home with our conflict agreement, I thought there might be a chance we could salvage our marriage. We stuck to the agreement faithfully for several weeks. Then our twice-a-week meetings, to talk about anything that was bothering us, dwindled to none. I kept asking to meet, and he kept putting it off. Eventually, we went back to our old behaviours. It was not long before tensions escalated again. I knew I could not live like that. I asked him to either go to marriage counselling with me or else we would need to separate. We went for one counselling appointment and it was clear to me there was nothing left to save.

I decided to see another counsellor on my own for a while. He specialised in addictions counselling. It was during a session with him that I said, "I think I know what I need to do, but I don't think that I can do it." Meaning, I knew I needed to leave my marriage, but the thought of putting my children through that felt like it was more than I could bear. The counsellor asked me what would happen if I stayed. I told him my soul would die. He asked me if I wanted to live and I said, "Yes." He said, "Well, then I think you know what you need to do." Keeping my marriage together was coming at the cost of selling my Self. Despite my earlier intentions to make it work at all costs, I now knew that was too high a price to pay.

I saw the counsellor in late fall. I did know what I needed to do, but the thought of tearing my family apart ripped my heart out. I wanted so much for there to be another solution. Every morning I wanted to wake up and discover it was all a bad dream and that none of this had happened. I wanted us both to be working together to save our marriage. But the reality of the situation kept reminding me this was not a dream. You could have cut the tension in the air in our home with a knife. We were living separate lives under the same roof.

Interestingly enough, in the midst of all of this, it occurred to me that life had found a way to bring me around to forgive another piece around my mother. What must it have been like for her to make the decision to leave my father and her children in order to save her Self?

I did not know what the fall-out from my separation would be, but the thought of not having my children with me full time was torture. I loved them more than life itself, and I did not want to cause them pain. Yet, when I thought about what I was teaching them by remaining in an unhappy relationship that was detrimental to me, I knew I was not walking my talk. The message I wanted to give them was one of love and forgiveness. I wanted them to eventually come to understand it was okay to stand up for what they believed in, that it was okay to take care of themselves, and that women deserved to be treated with dignity and respect. I tried to do that within my relationship, and it had not worked. I knew in my heart it was time to move on.

But I was not going to split up my family just before Christmas, so I waited to tell my husband. Then it was his birthday in January, so I waited some more. In the meantime, a friend of mine introduced me to Debbie Ford's book, *Spiritual Divorce*. I was so grateful for that book. It helped me to view my upcoming separation from a place of love rather than a place of fear. It also helped me to reframe a lot of things and focus on the gifts from our marriage, rather than the things that went wrong. Neale Donald Walsch wrote the foreword in the original edition, and in it he talked about the concept of relationships. My understanding of what he wrote was that relationships never end, they just change form. This was something that resonated with me, and something I held onto throughout the separation. I still loved my husband, and that feeling has never changed. I just could not live with him. It was early February when I finally told him of my decision. I do not think he was surprised, but I think he hoped it would not happen. I do not know how much longer he would have lived on in quiet desperation in the marriage. Maybe he was relieved I was taking the role of the 'bad guy'. I do not know if that is true or not, because we never talked about it. We decided to wait to tell the kids as it was Laken's birthday in February and Allison's in March. I felt sick to my stomach all the time and I cried a lot. This was the death of a dream for me. When the time came, telling our children was the hardest thing I have ever had to do.

We all lived under the same roof until the sale of our house closed on May 1st. This was trying emotionally for all of us. I wanted everything to be over and done with now, while simultaneously anticipating the separation with dread. Even though I knew this was what I had to do, there was a large part of me that did not want to let go.

During that couple of months I drew up and filed our separation agreement. Included in it was a co-parenting agreement I drafted stating we would co-operate in a co-parenting relationship that revolved around what was in the best interests of the children. Despite our differences, the children's needs had to come first. We divided up all the assets and paid off all of our debts. At the end of this process I ended up with enough money to put a down payment on my own townhouse. Negotiating a real-estate deal was a new experience for me. My husband always looked after that kind of thing before. Up until the time the sale closed, I still was not sure I could make a go of things on my own, but I knew Spirit was calling me on to something bigger.

Many new things happened for me as a result of our separation and subsequent divorce. Each time fear of the unknown would come up, and each time I moved forward in spite of the fear, I felt more empowered. I saw a lawyer when I was first considering what my rights were if I left the relationship. It was at that point I decided I did not want lawyers involved if at all possible. I had a couple of friends who divorced using a lawyer and no one seemed to win except the lawyer. My goal was to approach the dissolution of our marriage with as much love and co-operation as I could muster. Some days were easier than others. But as long as I kept bringing it back to love, I knew we all would be winners in this situation. My husband and I could go forward with our dignity intact and our children could only benefit from having parents who were not at each other's throats all the time. That energy of co-operation followed us through to our joint divorce application, and beyond.

I am not saying we did not have many challenges along the way. As I was stepping into more and more of my own power, our relationship needed to be continually re-negotiated. Sometimes I asked the question, "What would love do here?" one hundred times a day. My husband did not have the responsibility of taking care of the children on his own very often. With the separation he had them two nights a week and every other weekend. There was a steep learning curve for all of us. He needed to find his own way and I needed to let go of thinking it had to be done my way. The children needed to forge their own relationship with their dad without my interference. The greatest gift I could give my children during and after the separation was to find ways to love and respect their dad.

On the day the sale of our family home closed, my husband was the first to leave. The girls and I were upstairs when he came to say goodbye. We stood at the top of the stairs. First he hugged his daughters and then he and I hugged for the last time. I cried then as I am crying now writing this. Our parting was so not what I wanted to happen. I knew I could not stay, and yet it broke my heart to leave. My only hope was that, in time, our children would be able to see their father and I were happier on our own and this had to be. After everything was removed from the house I went around to every room and thanked it for the shelter and the warmth it provided for us in the time we were there. Then I went into the backyard and touched each tree and thanked it as well. There were so many things that made our house a home. I did not want to lose the feeling of home in the move.

I made a commitment to myself that I would not enter into another relationship for at least two years. Even though the ego part of me wanted to blame everything on my ex-husband, the higher part of me knew I had equal responsibility in the demise of the relationship. With him gone I would now have to stay in my own backyard, metaphorically speaking, and examine my own behaviour. It was not my job to try and change his way of thinking. The only person's thinking or behaviour it was my job to change was my own. I no longer had anyone else to blame for my unhappiness.

It became clear that one of the things I was not giving in the relationship was honesty around my feelings. How could I expect to have a close relationship with a partner if I refused to let him know those most vulnerable parts of me? Another big revelation came around the expression of anger. Or the lack of expression, as was the case for me. We all experience anger. By me not owning my own anger, I subconsciously chose a partner who would express it for me. Then I got upset with him for doing what I unconsciously set him up to do. I began to wonder how many other areas there were in my life where I was projecting my disowned stuff onto him, and to others. Those answers continue to find their way to me as long as I am open to receiving them.

I sent a letter to my husband in which I was able to express gratitude to him for all the gifts our relationship provided for me. One of those gifts was his financial support during the several years I was recovering from cancer. Even though I did not value material things anymore, I wanted to acknowledge how the money was a blessing, because it gave me the time and space to really delve into who I was. There were good things in our relationship too. I tried my best to recite as many of them as I could in the letter. What I knew for sure was I had deep gratitude to him for the gift of our children. They bring such love and light into my life, and they are two of my greatest teachers.

Tools for Transformation

- *Are there areas in your life where you are settling for the status quo? What action on your part would bring more of the Real you into the situation?*

- *What is your definition and measure of success?*

- *Where are you sure you are right? Can you open yourself up to other ways of seeing things in the middle of that?*

- *How much of your efforts are directed at changing someone else's thoughts or behaviours? Can you shift to changing your own thoughts and behaviours?*

- *Is there something you fear doing at the moment? What one step could you take towards that fear? Take notice of your feelings after you have taken the step.*

- *What life situations have offered you an opportunity to see a past event in a different light? Is forgiveness possible in this place?*

- *Are there some feelings, or parts of you, that you are not owning and projecting onto someone else?*

- *Which relationships in your life have changed form through divorce, death, or some other form of perceived loss? Are you able to tap into the essence of them, even though they have changed, and focus on the gifts they brought to you?*

16. Loving Self and Other Equally

"All parts of the Great Mystery's creation are made in wholeness. I honor the wholeness in me as I revere the perfection placed in all living things."

Jamie Sams

FOR MOST OF MY LIFE I HAVE had a distorted concept of love. There were very few instances in my childhood when love was given unconditionally. My experience was that the commodity we call love was usually bartered in order to get something in return. I will love you if you are quiet. I will love you if you make my life easier by doing what I want you to do. I will only love you if you meet my needs. I will love you if you follow the status quo. Do not rock the boat or I will withdraw my love. If I love you desperately enough you will love me back. As a society we have bought into these myths for the most part. How could we not have? We are bombarded with media images of it everywhere we turn. In magazines, television programs, books, and newspapers the message is the same. You are not okay the way you are. Buy this product, or look like this person, or aspire to this type of relationship, and we promise you love. The mindset seems to be that love is something outside of us and we need to *do* something in order to earn it.

What a futile journey that mistaken belief has taken us on. We spend years, sometimes lifetimes, and thousands of dollars searching externally for that which has been inside of us all the time. Real love is not a form of currency. We debase it by trying to use it as such. If love is not shared freely, without restrictions or expectations of receiving something in return, then it is not love. Real love is a part of who we are because we are connected to Source and to each other. We need not fear there is not enough of it, or that we will not get our share. Love is limitless. The only limits it has are the ones we place on it.

When we extend authentic love to another, we are in essence saying, "The highest part of me sees the highest part of you, and I greet you there." There are no "ifs" or "onlys" or "buts" in that greeting. It is a pure and simple statement of Truth. In that place we are able to witness and observe our lives and the lives of others with clarity, openness of heart, loving detachment, and compassion. There are no strings attached.

I am challenged sometimes in remembering the highest part of me is pure love. Yet I experience undeniable glimpses of it in moments of joy. When I looked into the eyes of my babies; when I am in tune with my body and with nature; and when I connect with another in compassion. In those heart-centred places there is nothing else but love. When I am not in joy, I have allowed fear-based thoughts to creep in and knock me off my centre. In those instances, once I regain my balance, I begin to examine my intent behind my thoughts and actions. If I am in fear, then somewhere along the line I have stepped out of love. At any point I can choose to step back in.

Most of the time I have been clear on whether or not I was offering real love and compassion to another. Where I often fell short was in offering myself an equal degree of the same. The equivalent of reserving the good china for when company came. This was programming from my past. My work continues to be recognizing I am also an honoured guest at the table of life. We all deserve the good china, every day. If I am not recognizing the love inside of me and living my life from that place, then I am robbing the world of my little piece of heaven on earth.

Before I could perceive my seat at the table, I needed to tap into that reservoir of love within me more often. I started by focusing on my strengths and personal resources and applying those to the areas of my life that were not functioning well. I gave some thought to the experience of falling in love. What a curious expression that is. Are we actually falling, or are we rising up to our greatest potential in that state? I began to recall the delicious euphoric feeling of being in love. I felt like I was on the top of the world in that place. I started to ask myself the question, "What would it be like to fall in love with yourself, warts and all?" I tried to imagine what that would look like, feel like, smell like, taste like, and sound like. I began to visualise that with all of my senses. If I recognised the love at the core of my being how would I treat myself in every moment? How would I romance myself? For me that looked like expressing gratitude for all the gifts in my life, respecting where I was at in every moment, feeding my body nutritious foods, exercising the temple that is my body, honouring my body's messages, feeding my soul through creating peaceful beautiful surroundings, listening to music, spending time in nature, meditating to connect with Source, buying myself flowers, affirming my Divinity consistently, and engaging in loving relationships with others. I was not waiting for, or expecting, anyone else to meet those needs for me. They were loving things I could do for myself.

This love also extends beyond personal and interpersonal relationships. In the quote at the beginning of the chapter Jamie Sams talks about the perfection placed in all living things. Not only are we connected to Source and to each other, but our energy also blends with all life force energy. What we think and feel and say and do has impact. It matters that we are here, and it is important we live our lives from that consciousness.

In my marriage and in many of my relationships I tried to overlook unloving behaviour from others in an attempt to avoid conflict. Not only was that not a loving thing to do for myself, it was also not a loving gesture to the other person. It taught them abusive behaviour was okay. It is not. We are all deserving of love, dignity, and respect. Loving self and other equally in this situation would entail setting healthy boundaries that considered the needs of all concerned. It is helpful to recognise the cry for love underneath what appears to be someone else's unloving behaviour. At the same time, it is okay to let them know, from your heart, how their behaviour impacts you.

Boundary setting is not about drawing lines in the sand and trying to change someone else's behaviour. It is about taking responsibility for your own feelings in the middle of any upset and communicating that from a loving place. You can then decide what actions are required on your part to look after you.

The chapter title talks about loving self and other equally. It could just as easily be called respecting self and other equally or considering self and other equally. This is a good equation in all areas of life. Gone are the days of win/lose interactions. Two of the concepts *A Course in Miracles* teaches are that our brother's/sister's interests are no different from our own, and that we all go home together. We are in an age of co-creation on our planet. This is a time of finding ways to work together for the betterment of all. Creating a more peaceful, loving world is only possible if you consider both sides of the equation in all your interactions...self and other.

All of my relationships are mirrors of the relationship I have with me. It is my responsibility to make that connection with my Self a loving one. What a different world it would be if we could learn to see ourselves the way those who truly love us see us. I think it is time we learned how to celebrate our Selves and the magnificent beings that we are.

Tools for Transformation

- *What is your experience of giving and receiving unconditional love?*

- *Do you offer Real love to yourself? If not, take one step today to demonstrate love to you.*

- *Describe what it would be like to fall in love with yourself? How would you romance yourself?*

- *Are you accepting unloving behaviour from yourself or another? How can you change that?*

- *How do you celebrate yourself? Make a list of 10 things you are proud of doing. Then make a list of 10 things you love about yourself. Post these lists somewhere in your home where you can see them. Continue to add to this list over time.*

- *Try the Self-Love Meditation in the Resource Section at the end of the book.*

17. Gratitude

"If the only prayer you said in your whole life was,
"Thank you," that would suffice."

Meister Eckhart

THE TRANSFORMATIVE POWER OF GRATITUDE found me after my breast cancer diagnosis. I touched on moments of appreciation throughout my life, but gratitude did not become a consistent practice for me until I received the not so subtle reminder that my life was a gift. The beauty of gratitude is that the house does not have to fall down around your ears for you to begin the simple practice of it in your daily life. No matter what shape your life is in, you can incorporate gratitude into it this very moment.

Gratitude does not require all sorts of expensive equipment; you do not need to belong to a club or an organisation to partake in it; and no one is going to judge whether or not you have done it right. It is not a spectator sport. All it asks of you is your commitment to spend a few moments visiting it every day. For me, gratitude began as a simple, sacred, private practice and then began to spill over into all areas of my life. It required that I move from occasionally appreciating the good things in my life to consistently acknowledging them in some way.

During my breast cancer journey I developed what I called an "attitude of gratitude". Rather than focusing my energy on the grisly side of cancer, I made a choice to appreciate the many wonders that surrounded me. I was appreciative of whatever time I had left. I am not saying I buried my head in the sand and went into denial. I allowed my feelings to come up, but I did not dwell on the negative ones. I made a conscious choice to remain in gratitude regardless of the external circumstances in my life. I may not have been able to control the quantity of days I had on the planet, but I certainly had the power within me to determine the quality of each day.

My practice of gratitude helped me to let go of the resistance I had to what was happening in my life and allow the energy of acceptance and harmony to take its place. I started keeping a gratitude journal. It was on my bedside table, and I wrote in it every night before I went to sleep. I would go over my day in my mind and then write down at least five things I was grateful for from that day. I began to recall those moments of Real life you cannot put a price tag on: the smiles of my children, the smells of springtime, the beautiful colours of autumn leaves, the tastes of summer cooking, hugs from a friend, laughter, and the sounds of life being lived in our home, to name a few. Some days the journal was filled easily with many things. Some days it was more of a challenge to find things I was grateful for. On those days I would write I was thankful for another day on this earth, I was glad the day was over, I was grateful for the roof over my head, happy to be able to sleep in my nice comfortable warm bed, and honoured by the gift of my beautiful children.

Eventually, I began to add another step to that ritual. When I woke up each morning I would make a mental list of five things I was grateful for. So, even before my feet touched the floor to begin my day, I was starting it from a place of love. From there I moved on to outwardly expressing gratitude wherever and whenever something happened that reminded me of the beauty of life. Sometimes that took the form of a compliment paid to someone in person or a letter of gratitude for a job well done. The opportunities for expressing and welcoming gratitude into my world were endless.

The more I embraced gratitude, the more things came into my life to be grateful for. I was beginning to understand that what I put out into the Universe came back to me in kind. I did not have knowledge or an understanding of metaphysics at that point. But I was experiencing the direct result of cause and effect. Applying the love-based energy of gratitude was raising my body's energetic vibration and attracting things of higher vibration to me. There were no random occurrences. I felt like I called everything into my life in order to grow. Things that happened were not inherently good or bad. They were just things. It was how I chose to view them that led me to label them one way or the other. If I used fear-based thinking and labelled them bad, I had one kind of experience. If I approached them from a perspective of love and labelled them good, I had a different one. I was not the victim of my circumstances after all; I was the creator of them. As I moved away from my fear-based thinking, my world shifted more and more towards peace.

Lastly, I expanded my gratitude practice to include people and things that really ticked me off. If I was willing to perceive events with an open mind and an open heart, I could see how all so-called negative people and experiences in my life gave me an opportunity to open my heart wider and increase my capacity for love and compassion. That love included self and other. I now look at the people that trigger me the most as a gift in my life. They are some of my greatest teachers. Whenever I am in reaction and am holding anger and unforgiveness in my heart, I know that some of the places in me I still need to heal have just been illuminated.

Children, life partners, and our families of origin are amazing as they serve in their capacity as lights into the dark spaces within us! They can push our buttons like no one else can because they are closest to us and know our most vulnerable places. Perhaps that is part of their job here. Some of my greatest learning and growth has come when I recognise my reaction in the moment is way out of proportion to what has just happened. Then I know it really does not have a lot to do with the present situation. The present has served as a flag to an unhealed area of my past.

I have learned to express gratitude for the large and the small miracles, and especially for the things that do not appear to be working so well in my life. I have faith there is a bigger purpose or a grander vision behind them than I am able to see at the moment. I ask respectfully for that vision and/or purpose to be revealed to me when it is in my highest good to do so.

Over the last several years I have refined my 'attitude of gratitude' into an 'attitude of gratitude and grace'. I am grateful for everything that appears in my life because I recognise the loving influence of Spirit operating through these things. I am moving towards reaching my highest potential through grace.

Tools for Transformation

- *What does gratitude mean to you? Do you practise gratitude on a regular basis?*

- *Begin a gratitude journal and write in it every day, listing at least five things you are grateful for.*

- *Before you get out of bed each morning, spend a few moments and think about five things you are grateful for as you begin your day.*

- *Pick an experience from your past that you may have labelled 'bad'. In retrospect can you see how the experience may have been a gift? Did it present you with an opportunity to open your heart, heal a past hurt, and/or forgive someone?*

18. Balancing Feminine and Masculine Principles

"We've come into the presence of the One who was never apart from us."

Rumi

ACROSS MANY DIFFERENT CULTURES and spiritual ideologies the feminine principles are often associated with intuition, creativity, receptivity, tranquility, water, Mother Earth, and the moon. The masculine principles are linked with logic, assertion, focus, fire, Father Sky, and the sun. These feminine and masculine attributes are processed predominantly by different sides of the brain, with the right side of the brain associated with the feminine aspects and the left with the masculine. In some eastern cultures the polarities of these energies are called yin and yang, with the yin energy representing the feminine and the yang representing the masculine. In Jungian psychology the terms anima and animus are descriptions of two archetypes of the collective unconscious mind. Anima is the unconscious inner feminine personality of men, and animus is the unconscious inner masculine personality of women. When I am referring to feminine and masculine I do not mean female and male in the biological sense. Women and men have both feminine and masculine energies within them. Although these principles appear to be opposite forces, they are actually equal complimentary energies that are interconnected and interdependent. When they come together in balance they make a greater whole that is stronger than its individual parts. One flows into the other and they transform each other within that dance.

Whether we are talking about the physical, mental, emotional, or spiritual realm, it is important to remember that the feminine and the masculine would not exist without each other. Each contains the essence of the other. They are like two sides of the same coin. We all

167

have both within us, and we have access to both through the collective unconscious. Problems result when we allow one energy to consistently dominate, at the expense of the other. Then we are out of balance. Our culture in the west has supported this imbalance. In my generation little girls were encouraged to play with dolls, express their emotions, not express their opinions, and wait for Prince Charming to come and choose them. Little boys were encouraged to play with cars and guns, be 'big boys,' not cry, express their opinions, and seek out their princess. Deviating from these roles often resulted in societal ridicule, shaming, rejection, or worse.

This has set men up to disconnect from their feelings, from themselves, from other men, and from the rest of the world. And it has set women up to deny their own power, to seek approval outside of themselves, and to believe they are somehow less than men. So our men are alone on isolated islands and our women are burning themselves out trying to prove they are equal to men, and that they can be everything to everyone. No man is an island and women were not meant to try to save the world on their own.

I believe healing will come at a personal and global level when men begin to connect with other men and the rest of the world at a heart level, and when women begin to remember their power comes from within and from Source. As women and men, we have very unique gifts to bring to the table and to offer to each other. These gifts are not more or less important. They are simply different, and all of them are necessary for a healthier world. Women appear to be a step ahead of men at gathering together in groups for mutual support. But often we have gathered together to complain, usually about men or about other women. I have made a conscious effort to stop perpetuating the negative. Instead, I search for and create groups of women who gather to affirm and expand on what is already great within themselves and in each other. From that expanded place in me, I can come together with the men in my world and teach them what it means to live from the heart. Then men, who are learning to connect, can feel welcomed home from their island because I have created a sacred space for them to come home to. In that environment they can feel more comfortable offering their gifts and teaching me to respect the masculine principles in them and in myself.

My heart goes out to all women. In our roles as caregivers and custodians of the heart of the world, we have often had a tough road to travel. We have steadfastly nurtured that soft place in humanity, even when half of the world has denied that it existed. Sometimes we have been beaten and burned at the stake for doing so. I also salute the men in the world. Their role has not been any easier than women's. They have traditionally been the hunter/gatherers and the protectors. Roles where they needed to hide their hearts because vulnerability would have been a liability. Now the world is calling for a shift in all of us. We are moving from an 'us and them' mentality to one of co-creation. Women are better prepared in their biology and their upbringing to understand the rhythm of life and to go with the flow. For the most part men have not been provided with the same tools to make that shift. They are learning by trial and error as they go along.

I have noticed within myself that my personal growth has involved owning both the feminine and the masculine energies within me. As a child I learned to disown the feminine because it was not safe, and I was ashamed of my mother who was my role model for femininity. I became a tomboy and nurtured more of the masculine energies within. As I got older and realised I was safe, I began to let more of my feminine energies come forward. Then I started to alternate between the two. More of my masculine energies took centre stage again after my separation and divorce. I needed to look after my children and myself, and I felt like I needed to be both mom and dad to my children when they were with me. Gradually I have relaxed my fear-based approach to being a single parent and in that letting go, more of my feminine energies have come forth once again.

We are usually dominant in one or the other principle at different times in our lives. Awareness is the key to not excluding one or the other in ourselves or judging them in others. If we are accepting of the feminine and masculine principles within us, they will come forward and recede naturally as they are needed in our day to day life.

One Is Not Better Than the Other – We Need Both to Create a Balanced World

As a species we have lived in a world dominated by the rules of patriarchy for at least the last 6,000 years. The structures of our cultural and political systems have been dominated by the masculine and for the most part have excluded the feminine. This has not been healthy for our planet or for our evolution as a species. We cannot move forward if we are leaving half of ourselves behind, or if we are judging ourselves or others. That applies on both an individual and a world level. I have witnessed things beginning to shift, and I am very grateful to be part of that shift. I am grateful for the pioneers in this endeavour. The generations of women who have refused to accept the status quo and stepped more into their power, often with great personal sacrifice. And the generations of men who have recognised that something is missing in the world and who have gone within and without to search for a better way.

We are a global community and living as a patriarchal society is no longer serving us. But a co-creative world does not necessitate a pendulum swing to a matriarchal society either. There is tremendous value in finding a balance between the two, a blending of the feminine and the masculine. Tapping into the feminine in ourselves and our world sparks innovation, dreams, connection, and compassion. Being in touch with our masculine energies helps us to focus and get things done passionately. The masculine gives things form; the feminine gives that form life. The feminine births possibility; the masculine gives that possibility direction and focus. We can use our heads and listen to our hearts simultaneously.

In the world of work outside the home, it is possible for women to bring more of their masculine energies forward without going to the extremes of emasculating men or steamrolling over other women. And it is possible for men to bring more of their feminine energies forward without fear of losing control and focus, or ending up in a puddle on the boardroom floor.

We can also apply these principles to our relationships outside of work. There is nothing more inviting than a woman who is standing authentically in her power, or a man who has allowed himself to be vulnerable. Balance is the key. All it takes is a little willingness and a lot of practice. Asking the questions, "What would love do here?" and "How do I love my self and other equally in this situation?" are a good start on this process.

Examining the feminine and masculine principles within my spirituality has posed an interesting dilemma for me for most of my life. Even though our family did not go to church, both of my parents came from Christian backgrounds. The area we lived in until I was 11 years old was predominantly Jewish, and we learned a bit about the Jewish culture in school. I attended a Mormon church sometimes with my grandmother when I was a young girl. I was exposed to the Muslim religion when we lived in Saudi Arabia, and I was in many different churches for friends' weddings, baptisms, and funerals. So I was exposed to a variety of religions, but none of them spoke to me. I loved many of the old churches though. As soon as I walked in I could feel the presence of God, but the messages that were being preached there did not reach me. How could they have when the language excluded me and the text implied that, by being female, I was less than?

I began to put together my own spiritual practice. I believed every religion had some redeeming qualities and there was not just one path to God. I chose practices from different ways of life that worked for me, and helped me to feel good about myself and my place on the planet. I practised my spirituality by being a living example of the values dearest to my heart: compassion, consciousness, love for all persons, inclusion, family, healthy relationships, nonjudgement, forgiveness, and integrity. They became the guideposts of my life. I practised with prayer and meditation and by walking my talk in all areas of my life. I began to see God/Goddess in the faces of my children, in the homeless person on the street corner, in the miracles of nature, and even in the people who robbed my home.

My walk with God/Goddess became a very personal one, and it was not attached to anyone or anything. The first time I read Neil Donald-Klotz's translation of *The Lord's Prayer* from Aramaic to English, it touched my heart in a way the prayer never had before. It began, "O Birther! Father-Mother of the Cosmos." Apparently Jesus' original prayer had not excluded the feminine when he spoke to his Creator. How could the Source from which we all originated not encompass both feminine and masculine principles? Receiving confirmation that Divinity was not exclusive opened up a whole new world for me that I continue to explore with a more open mind.

Once we reach a harmonious balance between the feminine and masculine principles in all areas of our life and in our world, we will own all parts of ourselves. Then we can move forward claiming the Truth of who we are. Men and women will be able to lay down their armour. We can leave the battlefield, hand in hand and heart to heart, paving the way for a whole new world.

Tools for Transformation

- *Are your feminine and masculine energies balanced, or do you notice you predominantly express one or the other? Was one or the other encouraged or discouraged as you were growing up? List some things you could do to bring these principles more into balance within you.*

- *To get in touch with whichever aspects you have repressed, try doing a visualization exercise. Sit quietly somewhere where you will not be disturbed. Close your eyes, breathe deeply, and relax. Ask to speak to whichever side of you is in the shadows (feminine or masculine). Ask it what it needs and how you can help. Then listen and act on the answers that come to you. Do this exercise fairly often until you feel you have begun to own this part of you. Then talk to both the feminine and the masculine and ask them to talk to each other to create a better relationship between the two.*

- *Do you create opportunities to connect with others in your same gender? If so, are these meetings positive and uplifting? If not, seek out support in groups that affirm and expand on what is already great within you.*

- *Does the religion of your childhood reflect who you are today? What or who is a God of your understanding? What spiritual practices would make you feel good about yourself and your place on the planet? Seek those out.*

- *What does practicing your spirituality (how you live your values in the world) look like to you?*

19. Connecting
to Mother Earth

"...our world is a sacred whole in which we have a sacred mission."

Joanna Macy & Molly Young Brown

I LOVE HOW INDIGENOUS PEOPLES FOLLOW the teachings and the rhythms of nature. They have a reverence for the perfect balance of feminine and masculine principles in the natural world. Their lives are intricately entwined, on so many levels, with that which supports them. They recognise everything contains Spirit, and they do not take from the Earth without offering her something in return. They understand the dependent relationship between all life forms.

I have been blessed to travel to many places on this Earth. In each location I have been astounded by the beauty, diversity, and gifts offered to me by this magnificent blue/green planet I call my home. Part of that has come from the amazing people I have met along the way, but the majority of it has come from having the eyes to see, the ears to hear, and the heart to feel the Great Mother's heart beating in rhythm with mine. Ours is a symbiotic relationship, and it sometimes feels like I have forgotten the feminine principles of compassion and connection with the rhythm of life when it comes to being a good steward of my Earth Mother's resources. The biological and ecological systems of our planet are one consciousness and I have been treating them as if they were separate: taking what I want, when I want, without giving thought to the deeper ramifications of my actions.

Nothing brought this home to me more clearly than the tragic oil spill in the Gulf of Mexico during the summer of 2010. As much as I would have liked to remove myself from any responsibility in that ecological disaster, I asked myself some tough questions. How many of the products I use every day are petroleum based? How can I change

175

that? Am I doing everything I can to reduce, reuse, and recycle so that the physical refuse from my daily life is not accumulating in landfills? When I go shopping, how many times am I making conscious choices that are good for the environment? Is my money invested in companies that have sound ecological practices? My answers to these questions showed me I am ecologically aware and making some conscious choices, but I still have a very long way to go to fully participate in healing the rift between humans and nature.

Even though I was thousands of miles away from the Gulf, I could almost hear our Earth Mother weeping. When I tuned in energetically I could feel the angst of those waters and the living creatures in them. At first I felt powerless, and then I began to remember the Truth of who I am. I was aware I was not alone in my grief. I went and sat on a log on the beach in White Rock, British Columbia and sent intentional healing prayers across the waters to the Gulf and to her inhabitants. I also sent healing prayers to the men and women who were trying to find a way to contain the spill. I moved out of the darkness of blame and sent loving energy to them. I believed the light of love would do more to solve the problem than the darkness of fear ever would. Then I gathered in groups to do the same thing with many other souls. My prayers and my intention to stay in a loving place felt in line with who I am. I realised that even my small efforts made a difference. I now understand at a deeper level how connected all life forms are and how sacred our home is. The Earth is the pulse of life and it is my anchor, keeping me grounded in this physical reality.

Grounding and Balancing in Nature

When I was a little girl I loved the water. I felt like I was home there. Whether I was on the water, in the water, or near the water, I felt a great source of comfort and connection with it. Nature in all of its many miraculous forms has served as a refuge for me throughout my life. Whenever I needed to feel grounded or yearned to feel part of something much larger than myself, I would turn to the Great Mother. As a child I did not know the reasoning behind my actions. I just knew it felt right, a homecoming of sorts. I felt held there, I felt supported there, and I felt like I belonged.

One of my favourite pastimes as a child was collecting rocks. I loved their colours and their textures and their permanence. I wanted to be a geologist and study those miraculous pieces of the Earth when I grew up. I wondered about their history and I was curious to know what they would say if they could speak. They were something solid I could hold onto in my world of chaos and uncertainty. At home, in my room, they served as a reminder of peaceful times; times of self-reflection and times when I understood at a soul level I was much more than a body. At a deep level they helped me connect to my essence. They held a timeless story in their make-up and yet they were so much more than their story. They were a small part of a much greater whole. Like all of us are. In the collecting of and connection to these treasures, I began to tap into my own inner wisdom without even knowing it, wisdom beyond my years that I was not consciously aware of. It took me many more years to really hear and have faith in that still small voice within on a consistent basis.

In my teen years, after my father's suicide and my subsequent move to Calgary, it was nature that again brought me back to Truth. When I looked out our apartment window at the Rocky Mountains in the distance, I marvelled at their majesty and their timeless beauty. They helped give me perspective on my problems. When I thought about how long they had been there, their permanence reminded me that human life is short in comparison. What may seem like an insurmountable challenge, in the moment, becomes a speck of time in eternity.

Throughout my life I have been moved by the wonder of the changing seasons, the flowers, the trees and the sound of waves crashing on the shore. The continuity in them all, and the life passages inherent in each. From the spring, new beginnings. Into the summer, a swelling and maturing into fullness. Then onto fall: the crescendo of sight and sound, a blaze of glory, a death of the old in preparation for the birth of the new. And finally into winter: the quiet, calm, restful time before the rebirth in spring when the whole cycle begins again.

It is interesting to me that all of the things in nature, that served to ground me when I was a child, continue to be a source of well-being for me now. No matter what is ailing me, going for a walk in nature brings me back to my centre. Stepping barefoot on the grass in the morning dew helps me feel the energy pulsing from the Earth. Being on or near the water soothes my soul. Witnessing the magnificent colours in a sunrise or a sunset, each one different than the last, reminds me of the uniqueness and continuity of all life. In my home I am surrounded by crystal pieces of the Earth that each have their own healing properties. When I am out in nature, or surrounded by her treasures, I connect with what is real and important and life affirming. Feeling and moving with the rhythm of the Earth connects me with All That Is. It helps to keep me grounded in the physical and be in touch with the spiritual at the same time.

Respect for Gaia - Learning to Treat the Great Mother with Reverence

Gaia is the sacred Greek Goddess who personified the Earth. What a beautiful name for our home. Gaia receives from all of us and from nature; she cleanses that which we give her and then she recycles it back to us in many ways that maintain equilibrium on the planet. There is absolute perfection in nature. Each element does what it has been called to do. A tree or a flower does not compare itself to another tree or flower and find itself lacking. It unabashedly delivers all of who it is in every moment. Each element also works together for the whole. Even in death, the shell of a tree's trunk and root system provides a nursery bed for new life. What a metaphor this could be for a human life well lived in service to the greater good of all.

178

There is simplicity in getting back to basics, to our roots so to speak. Within that simplicity lies peace, if we choose it. I am reminded of Henry David Thoreau and his two-year sojourn at a cabin on Walden Pond. He experienced the spiritual benefits of a simplified lifestyle during his time there. While part of me would love to go to a cabin in the woods for two years to do the same, I also recognise that the benefits of his spiritual discoveries are available to me every moment of every day. All I have to do is look out my window or step out into my backyard. On the days when I make time, there are many walking trails and bodies of water I can also choose to visit. If I am silent and reverent long enough in any of those places, Gaia will teach me everything I need to know about life. She is the ultimate guru because she is always available to mirror my perfection back to me.

If I consider each of my actions in that light, I am curious about the times I have taken my reciprocal relationship with Gaia for granted. She supports me; she sustains me; and she helps me connect to the core of my being. As in all authentic relationships, she does not belong to me. I am a guest here. I believe I need to come from a place of compassion and loving action in my thoughts, words, and deeds when I interact with my hostess. She is a living, breathing entity that works in concert with me. The very least I can do is be an aware participant in our connection.

Tools for Transformation

- *Do you consider yourself a good steward of the Earth's resources? If not, think of some ways you could change that. Each small step makes a difference.*

- *Are you ecologically aware and making conscious choices to preserve your home?*

- *What elements of nature help you to ground and find balance in your life? How often do you visit and appreciate them?*

- *Take one step this week to simplify your life by getting back to nature.*

- *While you are taking that step, set aside 10 minutes of that time in nature to do a meditation. Sit quietly and breathe deeply. When you feel totally relaxed begin to look around you. Something in your surroundings will catch your attention. Spend some time in communion with this object and ask it what its message is for you.*

20. Listening to
the Messengers

*"Pain and discomfort in the body, mind, and heart are
our physical, mental, or emotional bodies calling for our
attention so that we will attend to them."*

Michael Brown

WE HAVE BEEN GIFTED WITH INCREDIBLE TEMPLES to house our souls. Our bodies and all of their feedback systems, whether visible or not, continue to serve us until we take our last breath. I spent the first 35 years of my life taking my body for granted. Not only taking it for granted, but sometimes berating it for not performing or looking the way I thought it should. I was not even conscious that I was treating it with disrespect. It was almost as if I took over abusing it where my mother left off. My weapons of abuse were more subtle than hers; things like not eating well, not exercising consistently, weight gain, staying in unhealthy relationships long past when it was time to leave, and ignoring my body's messages. The results of my abuse were the same, though. I was telling my body and my Self I did not matter and I was not deserving of love and nurturing.

Breast cancer delivered a loud and strong message to me to WAKE UP! I had not paid attention to the whispers, the taps on the shoulder, or the two by fours over the head sent to me before that. I just found ways to get past whatever the crisis at hand was and then carried on as if nothing had happened. I was great at triage of others' hearts. I was so busy sorting everyone else's personal dilemmas that mine never even made it to the table.

What I discovered in searching out complementary therapies for cancer was that my temple consisted of four layers. There was the physical, the emotional, the mental, and the spiritual. I realised that in order to heal myself I would need to approach things holistically. All four layers needed to be cleansed and maintained if I hoped to experience peace and harmony in my life. There was no way around that. The only way was through, by going within. Some of the non-invasive natural ways I found to do that were: reading enlightening books, singing, nutrition, exercise, yoga, Reiki, counselling, self-development workshops, massage, cranio-sacral balancing, ThetaHealing™, EMDR, reflexology, iridology, bio-geometric integration chiropractic, massage, meditation, breathwork, family constellation work, healing laughter, and getting outside in nature, to name a few. I am sure there are as many avenues of healing as there are people seeking to be healed. It is important each person honour their own body's messages and do whatever works best for them at a pace that is comfortable. There are some methods that take you full speed to your walls and then push you through them. From my perspective this feels energetically abusive. Seek out healing and healers that are gentle on your body, mind, emotions, and spirit. Find things that challenge your way of thinking but allow you to make the choice about whether to move forward or not. Things that are respectful of you and your process.

The healing journey continues for me. It is like peeling back the layers of an onion. Once one layer has been shed, I get signs that let me know when it is time to approach the next layer. These signs come predominantly through my feelings, intuition, dreams, my over reaction in situations, and my body aches and pains. Sometimes they come directly from Spirit. The perfect book to illuminate my next step almost jumps off the shelf at me, or the perfect person to help me with the next layer appears in my life, or I am led to a gathering that speaks to my soul. Being mindful of all of my experiences increases my awareness of other external messengers that come in the form of animals that cross my path, or colours, or song lyrics, or others' conversations. All Spirit asks of me is to have faith and to trust in the process. The messages are being delivered to me all the time. My life runs more smoothly when I am open to listening. The nature of this journey we call life is to continually move towards rediscovering the amazing spiritual beings we are. The following are some of the feedback systems that send us messages to let us know whether or not we are on track in accomplishing what we set out to do in this lifetime.

Feelings

In my family growing up, my mother was mad, my father was sad, and all of us felt bad. I do not remember much glad. Feeling the whole spectrum of my feelings would have required me to move from my head to my heart. This was not a trip I had much experience taking in my younger years. Feelings got buried because it was dangerous to be in my heart. I needed to use my head to keep myself safe from the abuse. At least that is what the child part of me believed. I honour the child I once was. She did the best she could with the resources she had, and she helped me to survive. As I began reclaiming more of my authentic self as an adult, disqualifying my feelings no longer worked well for me.

The buried feelings might have been out of sight and out of mind, but they had not magically disappeared. They had, instead, become locked in my body and were causing dis-ease: my body's way of communicating it was not at ease. Our physical, emotional, mental, and spiritual essence is one of moving towards integrating all parts of ourselves. Feelings are a part of who we are. They are our body's indicators of what is going on inside of us. The natural state of emotions is energy in motion. The tremendous amount of energy it took for me to avoid, bury, and keep my feelings static and submerged left me with very little energy for anything else. I was, in effect, disabling my internal warning systems. I was subconsciously on guard all the time, and I was drained.

What I have learned is there is no such thing as a bad feeling. All of our feelings are valid. It is me who labelled them good or bad. 'Good' being synonymous with anything that brought me acceptance and 'bad' equated with anything that brought rejection or separation. Good or bad, sometimes the feelings were uncomfortable. Our culture has moved towards instant gratification. If it feels uncomfortable, mask it and get rid of it quickly. Some of us allow ourselves to feel the good feelings, but we try to disown our so-called bad ones. In my family home growing up, even the good feelings were squelched. It somehow felt disloyal to have any good feelings when my parents were so unhappy.

I found it was vitally important to embrace all of me, and that meant acknowledging all of my feelings. The decision then became, do I respond to the feelings or react as a result of them. Responding was a considered reply, as a result of looking into the impact of my actions, then expressing or acting on my feelings appropriately, if need be. Reacting was a knee-jerk reply that allowed my internal angst to spill out all over someone or something else. By taking responsibility for my feelings I learned how to feel them until they were integrated in me, instead of holding them at arm's length. They belonged to me. No one else made me feel a certain way and my actions did not cause someone else to feel a certain way.

Although it did not always seem like I had a choice in what I did with my feelings when my buttons were pushed, that is not actually true. In every moment I had choice. When I began to pay more attention to what was going on inside of me, angry feelings did not actually just appear instantaneously. They were often the result of little resentments that were building for a while. Rather than risk any kind of confrontation by examining or expressing the small resentments, I swallowed them and then they exploded, usually at the most inopportune times. I was into that extreme swing of the pendulum again, either under reacting by freezing and shutting down or over reacting by blowing up.

There was a middle ground. If I looked at anger as a wonderful teacher, I could see it had many faces. Sometimes it was a defense masking other deeper emotions I was afraid to tap into, and sometimes it was a signal my boundaries had been crossed. Oftentimes it was an indicator I had chosen a perception of a person or situation based on my way of seeing the world, which was not necessarily accurate. In any of these scenarios, anger extended an invitation to me to go beyond the surface and get curious about what was really going on for me.

When I examined my upset feelings, they were often connected to something I had not resolved from my past. If I could sit with them long enough and open myself up to their messages, they became windows into what I had buried inside of me. By looking at them that way, I could use present feelings to connect to past hurts and begin the process of unravelling them in the present. As I got more practiced at this I could sometimes anticipate what situations would be challenging for me ahead of time and begin to shift my perception before I entered into them.

Two examples of feelings that I have experienced challenges with are grief and joy. Dropping into the many levels of grief scared the hell out of me. I was afraid I would not be able to get back out. Grief has very patiently waited for me. When I did not grieve the losses from my childhood abuse, life found a way of helping me revisit them in parenting my own children. I did not fully grieve the loss of my father, so grief revisited me 20 years later with the suicide of a friend's grandson. I did not make time to grieve the losses associated with breast cancer and my mother's death because I had two small children to raise. That grief finds me now in quiet moments, in television shows and books that honour the paths of others who have travelled the cancer journey. As I allow these feelings to surface and move through me, I also open up a conduit to joy. What I had not realised was that holding back some of my uncomfortable feelings restricted the emotional flow that would take my life to the next level. I glimpsed moments of joy throughout my life, but it did not start to become a more constant companion until I was willing to feel everything. My feelings continuously give me opportunities to resolve my past. If I miss one chance, there is sure to be another just around the corner.

My dreams are the messengers for the feelings I have not worked through in my waking hours. Repeated dreams are a sign of something

I really need to pay attention to. They are communications from the collective unconscious. When I take time to decipher their symbolism, I am often surprised at how they bring deeper levels of awareness to me.

I am learning to move towards those people, places, things, and thoughts that feel good to me. And I am learning to not take myself and my life too seriously. Life is too short for anything else.

Intuition - the Still Small Voice Within

Out of all our messengers, intuition is the one that sometimes gets a bad rap. It is erroneously called "women's intuition," and it is often shrouded in myth and mystery, as if it is the exclusive right of a privileged few. It does not belong exclusively to women, but women often seem to be more in touch with it. It is predominantly a right brain activity. The concept of intuition seems to be largely dismissed by those not in touch with their feminine principles. If it cannot be quantified or proven scientifically, then for some people it does not exist. Even if we do acknowledge we have intuition, when it speaks, most of us question the validity of its messages.

We all have intuition. It is just a matter of tapping into it and then having faith in it. It is sometimes called the "still small voice within," with the operative word being 'still'. It was not possible for me to hear it if I was running around like a chicken with my head cut off. It gets lost in the din of mind chatter in my head if I do not make time for quiet contemplative moments in my life.

Intuition manifests for me as a gut feeling or an inner knowing that something is, or is not, for my highest good. It will also appear to me as goose bumps or an energetic tingling in my body. Sometimes I hear the messages as if a voice is speaking in my head. Many are the times I have ignored my intuition at my own peril. I cannot begin to count the number of unhealthy situations I have found myself in where I have realised in hindsight I did have intuitive warning signs I had not paid attention to.

Ignoring, discounting, or second guessing my intuition has a lot to do with control and ultimately with fear, on my part. I let my mind believe it knows what is best, and I try to make things happen the way I want them to. I attempt to orchestrate the events in my life so as to avoid chaos or vulnerability. Surrendering to the higher part of me, that intuition represents, can take me into the unknown. I have come to understand that even though the unknown can be scary, it is also the birthplace of possibility.

Another place I get stuck is in trying to interpret whether the voice is bringing messages from my higher self or from my ego. I trust that the voice is coming from my higher self if what it is asking me to do will ultimately bring more love into the world. Intuition is a powerful tool and a great messenger. The more I tap into it and use it, the more developed it becomes.

When the Body Talks

The mind likes to follow the path of least resistance regardless of whether it is for our highest good or not. Our bodies, on the other hand, do not lie. If I were to look back on my life, my body has been my barometer for my well-being. The problem for me has been whether I chose to listen to it or not.

When I was a child, I energetically left my body. It was the only way I knew how to survive the abuse. When I was a teen my body told me my dad was heading back down that black spiral of depression. I felt that lead weight in my solar plexus at the same time as my mind tried to convince me I was imagining things. In intimate partner relationships my body knows when the relationship is finished because I lose interest in making love long before my mind acknowledges our time together is done. Weight gain has often been an indicator that something is out of balance in my life. Rather than being a sign of excess, it is a flag to me of not enough self-nurturance. I have noticed I use the extra weight as protection. It has been a passive aggressive way to say, "Keep away from me." Breast cancer was my body's desperate cry for help. It was the culmination of years of shutting down my body's messages.

Our bodies are brilliant messengers and are talking to us all the time. If we are paying attention, there is a pretty immediate feedback loop. It is like a GPS system. When we are off track some part of our body will cry out for attention, in effect saying, "Excuse me, you might want to take another path. This one is not for your highest good." Louise L. Hay does a wonderful job of correlating the part of the body that is dis-eased with the possible message it is trying to send you in her book, *You Can Heal Your Life*.

I think it is important to remember when we have experienced emotional trauma that has not been resolved we stay stuck emotionally at whatever age we were when the trauma occurred. For instance, when my emotional buttons are pushed and some of my core wounds are touched on, I can revert to a six-year-old in a split second. Six was the age when I decided to shut down my heart and never let anyone in again. When we were little, if my mother found something broken or damaged and my brothers and I would not tell her who did it, she would punish all three of us. In this particular instance, I cannot even remember what she was angry about specifically, but we were all spanked and sent to our room. My brothers eventually cried themselves to sleep, but I would not let go of the perceived injustice of having been blamed for something I had not done. This was like the proverbial straw that broke the camel's back. Six years of being screamed at and hit and ignored were all being placed at the threshold of this one event. I lay sobbing on the hardwood floor of the bedroom in the dark, peering out through the crack of light at the bottom of the closed door. I was waiting for someone to hear me. I was waiting for someone to come and comfort me. I was waiting for someone to acknowledge the unfairness of it all. I waited a long time. I could hear my parents talking in the living room while they were watching television. I could hear my dad tell my mom she probably should go and get me. I could hear the silence of her lack of response. At some point in what felt like hours to a young child the door to my heart closed and locked. Not with a slam and lots of fanfare but quietly and sadly and resolutely. And no one heard.

From that one event I cemented into my mind some mistaken beliefs about myself: I did not matter, I was not lovable, and the Universe definitely was not a friendly place. I have done lots of work around correcting those mistaken beliefs, but there are times when the people closest to me in my life can still touch on deeper, unhealed layers of that most vulnerable place for me. Then my mind and my six-year-old take over the show. When this happens I know these are the places within me still needing to be healed.

If left unchecked, my mind will thwart my growth at every turn because growth often means change, and my ego perceives change as a threat to its survival. As soon as I started to step outside of my comfort zone in the writing of this book, the voices of the ego began their chorus of: "Who do you think you are? Shut up…no one cares what you have to say. Don't air your dirty laundry in public." It was really important for me to examine these voices and determine if they were speaking the truth. A good friend of mine has named these voices "The Committee of Assholes in My Head" otherwise known as 'The Committee'. 'The Committee' consists of the voices of generations past and of all the authority figures whose job it was to keep me in my place. It helped me at the beginning of my healing journey to think of them as assholes in order to be able to put some distance between me and the voices. At some points I visualised putting the entire 'Committee' into a boat and sending them out into the middle of a lake. On really bad days I considered blowing the boat up! This gave me breathing space to ask my body if the voices were speaking the truth. The contracted and sick feeling in my stomach would tell me they were not. Then I would ask to tap into my higher self to remind me what the truth was. I knew when I accessed my higher truth by the peaceful feelings in my body.

I do not call 'The Committee' assholes anymore. When I hear them I thank them because I know their messages were originally spoken by someone who was either trying to protect themselves or protect me from something 'bad' happening. Belonging has long been a method of survival and to go against the grain often meant death. Moving too far outside of what 'The Committee' deemed safe was all that was required to bring in the barrage of warnings. I remind them I am an adult now and can look after myself. What we resist definitely does persist. Acknowledgement and nonresistance of the voices helps me to silence them.

Meditation

This is one of the places where I make space for some of those quiet contemplative moments in my life. I shied away from meditation for a long time. It was a concept I really did not understand. I imagined you needed special training to do it, and you needed to spend hours every day at it. I allowed my fear of the unknown to stop me from looking into it for quite a while. The cancer centre in Toronto offered some wonderful complementary programs for patients to access during and after treatments. One of them was a weekly, one-hour guided meditation session. An hour felt manageable to me, so I decided to try it out.

The benefits were many. Just stopping long enough to relax for a few moments was worth its weight in gold. It deepened my breathing and opened me up to myself. It helped me to access that higher part of me where Spirit was able to deliver its messages. What I found was that meditation took me away from a state of doing and gave me access to a state of being. Afterwards I felt lighter energetically and physically. There were many forms of meditation. Anything that brought me into the present moment worked. It did not have to be a certain style or look a certain way.

For example, I can make dinner full of resentment at spending my time at such a mundane chore. Or I can use love and kindness and full awareness during every moment of the preparation. I can go for a hurried walk to get some exercise, while at the same time anxiously waiting to get onto the next task in my day. Or I can make each step during the walk a meditation of full awareness of the sights, sounds, and smells around me. I can choose to acknowledge the miracle of my body and feel the pulse of life within me. These are very different ways of experiencing the same events.

Have you ever watched ducks in a pond when they are not 'doing'? Their feet are completely still beneath the water and they drift in the current with ease. I do not know about you, but I prefer to go through life with ease and grace, not always caught up in the doing. I love feeling the contentment of simply being. Meditation takes me to that place. When I begin my days with even 5 or 10 minutes of meditation, I am more peaceful, calm, and surrendered to what is for the rest of the day. Then the goings on in the outside world have less impact on what is going on in my inside world.

Connecting to the Breath

Breath is life. It animates everything that lives. Finding this piece in my healing journey delivered me to some of the messages that were locked deep inside of me. I had not realised how constricted my breathing was as a result of my chronic childhood experiences of fight, flight, or freeze. Oxygen could not flow optimally to all parts of my body because my shallow breaths restricted the amount I took in. No wonder I was tired. It actually hurt to take a deep breath because my lungs and my rib cage were not accustomed to expanding that much. Most humans only use about one fifth of their lung capacity. I used even less.

As I started bringing my awareness to my breath I noticed there was a direct correlation between my shallow breathing and feeling tense. In those moments of anxiety, taking deeper breaths calmed me. If I made the time to take in three deep breaths and let them go with an audible exhale, I could feel the connection to my Greater Self, through the breath, in my heart centre. It brought me into present-moment awareness. This is something I can do for me no matter what is happening around me. Practicing this at least once a day, especially during the calmer times in my life, helped me to make deeper breathing more of an everyday occurrence. It was like a muscle, the more I used it the more developed it became. Then I was able to more easily drop into a relaxed present-moment experience, even when things were not so calm on the outside.

From regulating my everyday breathing patterns I was led to individuals and groups that taught more conscious connected breathing exercises I could use to tap into my emotional body. This is where my unprocessed emotional experiences from childhood were stored. Breathwork helped me to release them and begin the process of integrating them. Releasing the repressed emotional blockages in my body made way for joy to come bubbling to the surface as well. The good was buried along with the bad.

I now make a conscious effort to connect to my breath in all circumstances. If I am feeling overwhelmed it helps to ground me, and if I am feeling joyful the breath will help to anchor that in my body as well.

Tools for Transformation

- *What messages do you send your body and your Self by your actions?*

- *Have you tried any complementary therapies in balancing your life?*

- *If you changed your perception of your feelings and decided they were all 'good', how would that change your day to day life?*

- *What do you do with your feelings? What might be underneath your anger?*

- *Try keeping a dream journal. Look for the symbolism. Imagine each part in your dream is an aspect of you. What might those parts of you be trying to tell you?*

- *Do you use and/or have faith in your intuition? How does it present itself to you?*

- *What messages has your body delivered to you?*

- *List 10 things your 'Committee' tells you each time you step outside of your comfort zone. Beside each of the 10 things you listed, write whether it is true or untrue. For all the things that are untrue, re-write a statement that reflects the truth of who you are. If you have difficulty with this tool, ask for help from someone who loves you unconditionally, or imagine you are supplying these answers for your best friend.*

- *Try meditating for five minutes a day in whatever form suits you and your lifestyle.*

- *Try taking three deep breaths, followed by a deep exhale with a sigh, intermittently throughout the day when you are feeling overwhelmed.*

21. Excavating the Gifts

"If you change the way you look at things,
the things you look at change."

Dr. Wayne W. Dyer

THERE ARE A LOT OF CHOICES I COULD HAVE MADE in light of my past. I could have chosen to perpetuate the patterns of physical, emotional, verbal, and sexual abuse into future generations. I could have chosen to anaesthetise my pain with substance abuse. I could have chosen to be bitter about my childhood and lead a life full of anger and resentment. I could consider myself a victim and live my life from that place of negative energy. And sometimes I have. But I have found that a life lived in the moment, with joy and gratitude, is a more soul satisfying way to spend my time. It enriches my days and helps me to offer my best in the world. It brings quality to my existence.

Each of the events in my life has purpose and meaning. I do not believe in coincidences. My experience has been that everything I have called into my life has given me the opportunity to be both student and teacher in every moment. I can always choose my perception and response in all ways. Those whom I have viewed as my biggest adversaries could also be called my greatest teachers. By demonstrating to me who I am not, they have helped me to define who I am. By pushing my emotional buttons they have shown me areas of my past that I have not yet resolved. All of my experiences have opened me up to a more heart-centred way of living, when I have allowed them to.

By making the effort to look for the good that has resulted from things that could be thought of as negative events in my life, I have found it easier to make peace with my past. Without exception, each tribulation has come bearing gifts in its hands. I may not be able to see the gifts in the moment. Sometimes it takes years to see the benefits. But if I am patient, I begin to see how God/Goddess has orchestrated a Divine plan for my spiritual growth. Each piece of the puzzle falls into place when I am ready. I would not change one moment of my history because everything that has happened to me has helped to mould me into who I am today. I am really happy with me.

How to Shift Our Perception and Find the Gifts in Things Such As...

Abandonment

Even though my parents did not abandon me physically very often when I was a child, they were both so involved in their own pain they were unavailable to me emotionally, mentally, and spiritually. On the surface, abandonment appears to be inexcusable, and the thought of a parent abandoning a child brings forth all of our protective instincts. The word abandonment itself conjures up images of heartbreak and isolation.

While I do not deny I felt the heartbreak and the isolation, the flip side is that abandonment gave me the chance to get creative about looking after myself. I became resourceful and persistent. Forging my own way helped me to develop an entrepreneurial spirit and fostered independence in me. Realizing there was no one else to do things for me, I began to look within myself instead of being externally motivated. I tapped into my inner wisdom and relied on that in unfamiliar situations. This has been of tremendous value to me as I continue to learn to live in this world without getting caught up in its ego trappings.

The creativity I nurtured in my times of loneliness, led me to use art as a medium for connection and sharing higher Truths. The isolation led me to a lifelong love of learning, through the medium of books, and an appreciation of music. Developing the introspective part of me helped me to connect with nature, ground myself, and see my connectedness with all things.

Abuse

The experience of abuse helped me to develop inner strength and courage. Living through the most common forms of child abuse also gave me a heightened sense of intuition. I am a keen observer of people and situations, and I can sense energetically when they are not for my highest good. My experience of abuse also gave me an increased sensitivity to children who are experiencing abuse. I can read it in their eyes, in their energy, and in their body language. I see the hurt child in adults too, and energetically offer that inner child recognition.

Abuse was my biggest teacher of compassion. It helped me to come from a deep place of empathy in my interactions with others. It also helped me to develop unconditional love, for myself and others, and extend that out into the world. I can empathise with any living being who has experienced trauma. If they mistakenly believe they are irretrievably damaged, I can reflect the Truth that they are whole back to them. I have the ability to separate a person's behaviour from the Truth of who they are inside. I can see their potentially harmful behaviour as a cry for love and still send love their way.

Experiencing abuse brought forth a strong desire in me to stop its generational transmission. Having had all of my boundaries crossed repeatedly as a child, I am aware of not crossing that line with others. Because I have known the fear and found my way to the other side of it, I can be an example to others that there is hope in any situation. I can meet people where they are with nonjudgement and listen to them from my heart.

Addiction

Although addiction is frequently viewed as something negative, some of the reasons behind it are not. It is actually an ingenious way to self-medicate in order to feel or not feel. Problems result when the behavioural, physical, and emotional side effects of self-medication become damaging to our relationships with ourselves and others.

Most people I have met who are experiencing challenges with addictions are extremely sensitive to the world around them. They are, in their own way, seeking Spirit, the God/Goddess that dwells within them, but conducting the search outside of themselves. This inevitably leads to disappointment, and the addictive substance or behaviour is called in to soothe that hurt. Sometimes we are so bombarded by the constant frenetic pace of the world that we numb our senses to survive. Addictions in this instance can be used to help us feel something.

I have had my own addictive struggle with food most of my life. It was my drug of choice and I have used it in both of the ways described above. It has also been a source of comfort and a source of safety. I have mostly used it as a crutch so that I do not have to express my feelings directly to people. Food and I continue to re-negotiate our relationship. The only thing that works consistently for me in regulating my use of food is learning to love myself. As I go within and connect with that still small voice, my cravings for food decrease. Addictions let me know when something is out of balance in my life. My desire for food, when I am not physically hungry, alerts me that there is some other hunger not being satisfied. My job is to decipher what that hunger is and find a healthy way to meet that need.

Suicide

My father's suicide rocked my 18-year-old world. Some of the gifts inherent in it were evident fairly quickly. Others took over 30 years to come to light.

The loss of my father in such a tragic way brought my brothers and me closer together immediately. We took each other for granted before that. Losing our father so unexpectedly brought home to us that life was finite and it was important to cherish our time together.

Trying to rationalise why my father caused his own death started me down the path of questioning the deeper meaning of life. I began to explore an existential philosophy. What was I here for? What was the highest goal I could aspire to? What was the value and meaning of life? Could my father have made another choice? What could I do differently in my life to consciously shape it into one of purpose? I did not have the answers but at least I began to ask the questions of myself. I started to let go of the small stuff and began to see that only love matters. I do not remember the last thing I said to my father. I hope it was, "I love you."

As a result of experiencing the suicide of a loved one I am not scared off by people who are considering suicide. Some of them have told me I am a life preserver. I am not inhibited when they talk about their feelings with me. I can travel with them in the stormy waters without feeling like I am drowning. I would not consider suicide as an option for myself because I have witnessed first-hand the long-term emotional toll it takes on the people left behind. Removing this as a possible solution to my problems forced me to seek other avenues of resolution.

The most recent gift that has come to me from my father's suicide happened in the last few years. A good friend of mine asked me, "What do you need to teach that your father forgot?" My father forgot he mattered, his life had purpose and meaning, and no situation is devoid of hope unless you make up your mind that it is. I now go into local high schools and speak to teens to let them know they matter and to offer them hope. All of my work in the world focuses on this important theme.

Illness

My major illness was cancer, but I had lots of other childhood illnesses. I have also been a witness to friends and clients who are battling a number of different dis-eases of the body, mind, emotions, and spirit. Even though the symptoms of dis-ease may present themselves in different forms, the underlying message is similar. Our spirits are calling to us asking us to go within and pay attention to them. The messages they bring are specific to us and our life journey.

At some point in my cancer experience I stopped looking at the journey as a battle and my body as the enemy. I started to view my body as a very dear friend and the journey as a door to my feelings and an opportunity to clean up my past. It helped me to use the feelings stored in my body to find my way home to my authentic self. Cancer was my invitation to live a more conscious life of integrity, passion, and purpose. It taught me how to value giving and receiving love, over material possessions. And it gave me a huge wake-up call about listening to, and trusting, the wisdom of my body. It was my initiation into the mind-body connection and the power of my mind.

Cancer gave me so many gifts. The greatest gift was the reconnection with my mother. I do not know if anything less drastic than cancer would have shaken me to the core of my being and forced me to reevaluate my life. It gave my mother and me a common bond and helped us cut through all the crap from the past, to get straight to the heart of the matter. Life was too short to hold onto unforgiveness. I lived one of *A Course in Miracle*'s daily lessons: another's interests really were no different than my own. My mother and I could only find our way home together. We were not separate on the path.

Cancer also gave me an appreciation for all that was good in my life, an 'attitude of gratitude' for the things money could not buy. It helped me to say, "No," until I learned how to say it for myself. It was the start of my education on self-care. There were many people who came forward to help me. My transpersonal perspective on life really blossomed during this phase. I got, at a soul level, that there was more to life than the narrow perspective I had on it before. I was part of a bigger whole and the Universe really was a friendly place.

I learned a lot about perception and about reframing negatives to positives throughout my cancer experience. I even began to call the scars on the side of my breast and under my arm "catalysts for change". That was a much more positive reminder of the infinite possibilities in my life each time I looked in the mirror. Cancer enabled me to move from receiving healing to giving healing. I learned so much about complementary healing practices that I wanted to pay it forward and pursued a career in the healing arts as I began to regain my health.

Divorce

I am an advocate of trying to work through challenges in relationships. But sometimes the point comes when you realise your physical time together is done. Although divorce was the last thing I wanted to happen to our family, it gave me a new view on, and a new way to be in, relationship.

I learned to use cut-off and distance in my family of origin as a way to deal with conflict. But my husband and I had children together and that changed things for me. I committed to being the best co-parent I could be after the divorce, so cut-off and distance were not an option. I wanted my children to have their father in their life. To do that, I needed to find a way to be in a respectful relationship with him, despite the differences in our values and our approach to life. This change on my part was originally for the benefit of the children and ended up being for the benefit of us all. We were always going to be in relationship. The love between us had not died as the relationship shifted. The relationship just took another form.

Divorce opened up a path for my daughters to forge their own relationships with their dad that would not have been possible with me running interference in the middle. It showed me where I was over functioning in my marriage and in my children's lives and where I was under functioning in my own life. As long as I was busy trying to clean up what I perceived was a mess in someone else's backyard, the mess in my own was left untended. The more I worked on my own problems, the fewer problems I experienced with my ex-husband.

Death

I used to think of death as the final chapter. But I have had so many experiences that are telling me something different now. It is the closure of one chapter, but it is also a place of beginning the next step, or the next phase. Death, and the grieving process that follows it, applies to many life transitions. Full acceptance of the new requires relinquishing the old and the attachments we have to it.

Life is about growth in its many forms. As I came to believe Pierre Teilhard de Chardin's words, "We are not human beings having a spiritual experience. We are spiritual beings having a human experience," my response to death began to change. It is the release of one form to make way for another. It is my unwillingness to let go of the old that sometimes causes me pain.

As far as physical death of the body goes, we are so much more than just a body. We are an eternal spirit. Even though my parents are no longer with me on the physical plane, they are with me always in spirit. I now know angels on the other side of the veil.

Death serves as a reminder of the gift and the fragility of life. It has taught me to not take people and things for granted. My time is one of the most valuable gifts I can give to someone, and it is so important to be fully present when interacting with another. This moment may be all we have with each person we meet. I do my best to make each encounter a loving one.

Tools for Transformation

- *Is there anyone in your life who has helped you to discover who you are by showing you an example of who you are not?*

- *Can you uncover the deeper meaning in the messages of your dis-ease?*

- *Have there been times when illness is meeting some unfulfilled needs in you? Is there a healthier way to meet those needs?*

- *Can you identify some experiences of adversity in your life? For each experience, see if you can dig deep enough to find the gifts in them.*

22. Remembering the Truth of Who You Are

"The important thing is not to think much but to love much;
and so do that which best stirs you to love."

Teresa of Avila

THE NATURE OF WHO WE are is so much more than most of us even dare to imagine. I grew up believing I was inconsequential and God, if there even was a God, was some entity outside of me. I did not stop to think of the impact my actions had on others because I was not aware I had any impact at all. I spent a lot of years in that limited space. It is easy to see how that happened. I believed the external negative messages with which I was bombarded on a daily basis, not only from my mother, but from the media as well. Our consumer-driven society profits from our believing we are small and imperfect.

I AM As You ARE - Love and Light

I cannot identify the exact point when this began to shift for me. I know for sure that journeying through cancer certainly brought it to the forefront, but I would suspect my awakening was happening in gradual steps since my father's death. The birth of my children took things up another notch. When I looked into the eyes of my babies I saw love and light and perfection in them. And I saw God. If all of that was there in them, it must have also been there in me. I wondered when I lost it. Then I started to realise I had never lost it. It was there in me all the time. It was just covered up with layers of fear and darkness and perceived imperfection.

My personal growth work became about clearing through those layers of untruth and getting back to the core of innocence at the centre of my being. Love was my natural state. It was there, whether I could see it or not. I liken it to seeing the mountains in British Columbia. We have rainy and cloudy days where the mountains are not visible. My inability to see them does not negate their existence. Our innocence is the same. It remains untouched, no matter how many thoughts to the contrary we pile on top of it.

The pilgrimage to the light inside of me required that I cast myself as the hero in my own story. This seemed like a tall order in the beginning. Each step I took, with the intention of love, became easier. There could be no more waiting for someone or something outside of me to make me feel better. That had to be my job. I was the expert in my own life, and I had been giving away my power to others. My power lay in going within, asking questions, trusting the answers I received, and then acting on them. The first and most crucial step was for me to stop any self-negating thoughts, words, and behaviours. They were not serving me, and they certainly were not serving the world. The more I acknowledged the Truth and beauty of who I was, the easier my life became and the better I felt. The next step was to stop looking outside of myself for confirmation I was on the right path. I had all the tools within me to determine that. My feelings were my number one indicator. If I felt good about what I was doing, I was not only raising my energetic vibration but I was also helping to raise the vibration of the planet. Lastly, as I uncovered more and more of the love and light at my core, I needed to allow that love and light to shine in service to others. I needed to walk my talk in all areas of my life.

When I began this journey it felt like I was on the road less travelled. But the more I lived my Truth the more I discovered like-minded souls on a similar path. Sometimes along the way people moved out of my life. I allowed myself to feel the sadness around that, and then I blessed them on their way and released them. We are all Divinely created beings, but not all of our life paths are the same.

We are connected at a heart level to All That Is. We are love and light. We are home to the spark of Divinity placed there by our Creator. Mother/Father God and I/You are not different. We each contain elements of the other. I like to use the metaphor of the ocean, where God/Goddess is the ocean and we are the drops of water in that ocean. We are interrelated, interdependent, and part of the same whole. That spark of Divinity is not just in some of us. It is in every one of us. We do not need to do anything to earn it or to deserve it. It is ours by virtue of our existence. Our job is to remember it and tap into it on a consistent basis.

We Are All Connected

We are connected because we all contain that same spark of Divinity from Source. We may look different, but the core of us is the same. No matter what our race, religion, gender, or sexual orientation, we are all one. The illusion of separateness is just that, an illusion.

Contrary to my beliefs growing up, my existence is not inconsequential, and I do impact others. My thoughts, words, and deeds each hold an energetic vibration. Thoughts held consistently eventually become things. We are energy beings and our energy field extends out all around us. As we are going about our daily lives our energy is continually mingling with the energy of everyone and everything else. It is drawing from and contributing to the collective unconscious as well. What we think and say and do makes a difference, both in our little corner of the world and in the world at large.

There have been many theories posed that talk about this phenomenon. One is the "butterfly effect," where it is said that a butterfly flapping its wings creates tiny changes in the atmosphere that ripple out like a domino effect to potentially change weather patterns thousands of miles away.

There is also a story about the "hundredth monkey effect". It recounts how scientists, studying monkeys on a Japanese island, taught the adult monkeys how to wash sweet potatoes before eating them. Gradually the younger monkeys began to imitate the older monkeys and a new behaviour pattern was formed in the group. The fascinating part of the story states that once a critical number of monkeys were engaged in the new behaviour, in this case the so-called hundredth monkey, the new learned behaviour instantly spread across the water to monkeys on nearby islands. These monkeys had not received the training from the scientists or witnessed the new behaviour from other monkeys. It was transmitted energetically. There is controversy about the scientific proof of this story. But no matter how you choose to look at it, this is a beautiful parable about the possibility of affecting positive change energetically in the world.

Taking responsibility for our part in humanity's evolution requires that we do our own work to clean up our past and become conscious of how we use our energy to co-create in the present. In every moment we have a choice to become aware of our energetic connection with the rest of the world. I continually ask myself if my thoughts, words, and actions are spreading more love on the planet or more fear. If it is the latter, I change them.

Tools for Transformation

- *Are you able to see the spark of Divinity within you? If this is a challenge for you, can you see it in your child or in a beautiful, wise friend? In your heart, hold the possibility that what you see in others you also possess within yourself. What layers of untruths might be covering up that spark?*

- *Make a conscious effort this very minute to stop self-negating thoughts, words, and behaviours. If you do not have something good to think about, say to, or do for yourself…find something!*

- *How do you determine if you are following the path for your highest good?*

- *In what ways do you shine your love and light in service to humanity?*

- *To feel the energy field that surrounds you, try holding your hands with palms facing each other about one centimetre apart. If you concentrate on the sensation between your hands you will eventually begin to feel the energy moving between them. You may feel it as pulses, or heat, or vibrations, etc. Once you can feel this energy, begin to slowly move your hands apart in increments. Try two centimetres and feel the energy again. Then try three centimetres, and so on. Keep increasing the distance between your palms and notice when you are no longer able to feel the energy. This by no means indicates the extent of your energy field, it merely shows you your capacity for sensing energy at the moment. Then begin to move your hands back together in increments noticing the sensations again. Play with this. You can even try it with others. Notice how close others have to be for you to be able to sense their energy. Try doing this with your eyes closed and see how close another can get to you before you sense their presence.*

- *Have you ever had an experience of thinking of someone and then the phone rings and it is the person you have just been thinking about? Or been so in tune with someone else that you know what they are going to say before they say it? Take note of experiences in your life that show you are connected energetically with the rest of the world.*

23. I Am the Creator
of My World

"At the center of your being you have the answer;
you know who you are and you know what you want."

Lao Tzu

IT WOULD BE MORE ACCURATE TO SAY I am the co-creator of my world. Not only does that mean I am accountable for my part in creating the life I want, but it also means I am not alone. I have other souls on the planet who have agreed to accompany me in this lifetime, and I have unseen guides and helpers with me always. I need only ask for their guidance and help and then pay attention when it comes to me. Then I need to show up in the world by radiating the highest and clearest vision of who I am.

Just as I am accountable for the physical refuse I create in my life, I am also accountable for my emotional refuse. I need to be aware of what I am putting out into the world in the way of energy. The Law of Attraction gives me back what I extend. Fear and hatred only breed more of the same. If I want to create a life of more peace, love, and joy, then being and extending peace, love, and joy are what I need to focus my energy on.

Seeing the beauty in every facet of my life is a good start on that creation process. Believing there is a greater purpose behind all of the happenings in my life is another. So is blessing others, in all circumstances. To not do so is to hold myself apart from others with the mistaken belief that I am separate. That is not the way I choose to walk in the world.

Affirmations

Using positive affirmations is a simple tool that has transformed my life. They deliver a huge return for a relatively small amount of time invested. You can improve your health and bring more joy and passion into your days. Affirmations are positive statements you create, that affirm what is already true about you (whether you are able to see it yet or not), and about the vision you are creating for the life you desire and deserve. To be most effective, they must be framed in the positive and in the present tense. Then you need to repeat them consistently. If you repeated each affirmation 10 times and did that even as little as once per day you would begin to see your life improve.

Affirmations work at a number of different levels. They help to change your thoughts and increase your energetic vibration. As you think better thoughts about yourself and your life, you begin to speak more positively about both, and attract more of what you want into your life. Focusing on your vision and the feeling states surrounding it, while repeating positive phrases about it, begins to change your perspective.

The first step in creating affirmations is to spend some time thinking about the areas of your life you would like to improve. Make a list of these areas and then write a few positive statements for each one. For instance, if I wanted to create more peace and harmony in my life, some affirmations might be: "I am at peace." Or "I am calm and composed, and I have faith in perfect timing." Another good one that works for many areas is, "I love and accept myself completely." Notice how they are framed in the positive, and they are in the present tense. You can repeat them to yourself quietly, or say them out loud. You can also write them out or speak them in front of a mirror. Another effective way of utilizing them is to record them and listen to them as you are going to sleep each night, or create a screensaver for your computer that has your affirmations on it.

Affirmations are a way of changing out-dated behaviours and mind chatter, and replacing them with something positive that serves you. As in all things in life, the more you put this into practice the more you will get out of it. Doing it consistently will yield much better results than sporadic attempts. But even sporadic attempts are of benefit!

Creating a vision board is a visual and sensory form of affirming the life you are creating. A vision board can be something as simple as images and words, that represent parts of your dreams, cut out of magazines and pasted on a piece of poster board. Or it could be something as elaborate as painting your vision on a wall in your home. However you choose to capture your dreams and make them visible, will work. The key to activating the images and words on the vision board is to stand in front of it at least once a day and visualise yourself already living your dream. Imagine it with all of your senses: what does it feel like, look like, sound like, smell like, taste like, as you are living this dream? Create affirmations to go with the pictures and repeat those out loud as you are standing in front of your vision board. In this way you are sending out energetic vibrations that are a match to your dream and that will begin to draw the pieces of your dream to you.

How to Be the Change and Create the World You Choose to Live In

I had to get clear about what I wanted in my life. Sometimes that meant experiencing what I did not want first. Once I knew what I wanted, I began to release the things in my life that did not reflect that. Then I started to cultivate friendships and experiences that mirrored my higher vision.

I do not know of anyone who got to the point of experiencing peace consistently while hanging out and participating in chaos or negativity. I am not saying that 'stuff' does not happen in life, because it does. What changed for me was my perception and response to the 'stuff'. I used to believe that someday I would have done all of my personal growth work. At that point I thought I would have it all together and I could live in peace because challenging events would not happen anymore. I had set myself up to live in 'someday,' a kind of limbo land between now and never. While I was waiting for someday, I was not living my life today. I have come to understand 'stuff' will always happen, but I can choose my attitude, my perception, and my response in any circumstance. I have stopped waiting for someday to live my dreams. There is no someday to get to. There is only now. I do my best to live my dreams now instead of waiting for conditions outside of me to be different so that I can expand and grow.

Creating the world I want to live in required that I learn how to dream big. *A Course in Miracles* states that we do not ask God for too much. We actually ask for too little. I had allowed my horizons to be stunted by a society that felt more comfortable when everyone was in their place. Here is a beautiful affirmation from Alan Cohen, author of *A Deep Breath of Life*, "I move beyond my past and claim a glorious future. I manifest magnificent results because I think unlimited thoughts." Once I began taking one step every day towards my dreams, I brought more fun into my life which led to more joy. My days began to change for the better. Even if that step was as simple as dreaming about my dream and imagining what it would be like to live it with all of my senses, that sensory experience was enough.

There was a certain amount of *doing* involved in manifesting my dreams, but it was not what I was doing that defined me. It was who I was choosing to *be* in the middle of the doing that made the difference. I have been a spiritual counsellor in every job I have ever done, regardless of what form the job may have taken. I once worked as an administrative assistant and bookkeeper for a company that sold commercial greenhouse equipment. The office was located in an industrial complex in a fairly remote area. I cannot count the number of people who wandered into the office, off the street, and then stood before me and told me their life story while I listened with my heart. Once they relayed their story, they left, and I never saw them again. My boss used to just shake his head and say, "How do these people find you?" They found me because the experience I was seeking and giving in the world was a one-on-one heart connection. I can do that anywhere.

If I want to see and live in a whole, peaceful, joyful world, then I need to foster wholeness, peace, and joy within myself. This requires that I see and accept the perfection within me. It also asks me to follow my dreams. From that state of imagination and contentment, I can begin to witness the perfection in others. I can be the change I would like to see in the world. Peace anywhere begins with me.

Tools for Transformation

- *Are you aware of the unseen helpers in your life? How often do you ask for their guidance? Are you open to receiving that guidance when it comes?*

- *Write out 5 affirmations to help you create more of the life you desire and deserve. Remember to frame them in positive words and in the present tense. Find the way that works best for you to be able to repeat each affirmation 10 times per day.*

- *Create a vision board.*

- *If money was no object and you could be doing anything right now, what would it be? Think about what feelings you would be experiencing in the middle of that (i.e. peace, joy, love). What can you do in your life right now to create more of those feeling experiences you are seeking?*

- *What one step could you take today towards your dreams?*

24. Charting a New Path

"In all that you say, in all that you do, may nothing but light be surrounding you.
And peace in your thinking and peace in your dreaming.
And peace in your speaking, may peace be the tone.
Of each waking moment you spend here on this earth.
May peace be your vision until you find home."

From the song *Lady Lavender*,
written by Denise Hagan

EVERY ONE OF US IS A PERFECT MIRACULOUS MANIFESTATION of the Divine. We are not meant to be cookie cutter versions of each other. We all have unique gifts that only we can give. Being authentically us comes from within us. Our job is to get out of our own way and let those gifts come through, uncensored by conditioning of the past. The only limits we have are those we impose upon ourselves. If we allow it to, the magnificent Universe will deliver our wildest dreams to us. That allowing will come about as we heal what needs to be healed within us, align with the forces of light, and expand with joy into our full potential. There is no better time for that to happen than now.

As one door in life closes, another door opens. What you bring to the threshold of every door is what you have learned thus far about you. Each time you have the courage to step through an open door and enter into the unknown, you let the Universe know you are ready and willing to receive more pieces of the Truth of who you are. You gain access to your Greater Self as you move towards recognizing your own wholeness. Your prime relationship is with that Self. All other relationships will stem from that. Listen to the heart call from your Greater Self. When I tapped into mine this is the message it had for me:

June 26, 2010

Thank you. I love you.

You are amazing, a glorious human being. I would be grateful if you would visit me more often. I am your sacred heart and the place for you to hear your highest guidance. Sit with me in the silence. Sit with me in the serenity. Sit with me in the peace. And come to me when your life is not in harmony and balance. I have wisdom to share with you. I have love to share with you. I have grace to share with you. Come to me to remember the Truth. Come to me to tap into your Divinity. Come to me. I am here all ways waiting to join with you, with unconditional love and compassion. You are love. Remember that and remember me.

Love,

Your Sacred Heart Centre

Be the Truth of who you are unapologetically in every moment in order to flow with life. You will never be done exploring the many facets of who you are, and you cannot go wrong as long as you keep moving towards what is in your highest good and what is in the highest good of all.

Forgiveness - Transforming Quality of Life

Forgiveness of self and other is one of the cornerstones of peace, followed closely by surrender, trust, and faith. Forgiveness was one of the hardest pieces for me to get. We broached the subject in the Adult Children of Alcoholics counselling group I participated in. At that time I was adamant there were some people, and things, that could not be forgiven. I was still heavily invested in holding onto the story I told myself about my life, because that was how I defined myself.

What I did not understand then was that forgiveness was not about excusing someone's behaviour. It was about seeing the core of innocence in everyone. The events of my life had no meaning in and of themselves. The only meaning they had was the one I gave them, based on my perceptions. We see things through the filters of our past conditioning unless we make a conscious effort to do something different. Change begins with the awareness that things are not always what they seem on the surface.

A Course in Miracles (ACIM) defines everything in terms of it either being love, or a cry for love. When viewed from that perspective it is easier to see the innocence in another. My mother's and great-uncle's abuse of me did not mean anything about me. The only meaning it had was the one I gave it, namely that I had no value. Their behaviour was a cry for love. Underneath their exteriors were people who also suffered. I do not need to know the details of their suffering. I just need to remember it is there and honour it. As long as I carried unforgiveness of them in my heart, I carried the pain with me all the time. The abuse ended more than 30 years previously. I was the one still carrying it around. With forgiveness, I started out to set myself free and ultimately ended up setting all of us free energetically. Now our connection is one of love and compassion. Forgiveness ended up being a gift to us all.

The seeds of forgiveness were planted in me, first with experiencing the innocence of my children at their birth, and then with my perception around parenting shifting as I became a parent. Then those seeds were watered with compassion when my mom and I experienced breast cancer simultaneously. They began to flower as I looked into my family history and got a glimpse of some of the losses the family had not grieved.

My daughters and I took a trip to Ontario and visited the small hamlet where my mother's family's farm was. My mother grew up in that hamlet, my parents were married there, and I was sexually abused in the old farmhouse. We went to see the church first. It had not changed at all since the last time I saw it 30 years before. Across the street from the church was the community graveyard. There I found the headstones for my mom's family. Permanent markers to identify lives lived. By looking at them, no one would have known the amount of hurt and pain carried by the family. My great uncle's headstone identified he lived to be 99 years of age and never married. I was somewhat surprised he lived so long because he was dead to me from the moment I cut-off from my mother's family in my early teens. My daughter, who knew the stories of the abuse, said, "I think you should spit on his grave mom." I knew I had healed when I had no desire to do so.

After we left the graveyard, we drove down the road and past the old farmhouse. It had burned to the ground. All that remained were the four cement cornerstones of the foundation. The farm looked much smaller than I remembered it as a child. Seeing it presented a beautiful metaphor to me. I was putting my past in the past and starting from my foundation to rebuild my life. All of the old was burned away, and my past was no longer significant in determining my future.

What I discovered was forgiveness did not need to be shared with the person I was forgiving, for it to be effective. In the case of my mom, I did share it because I felt it would be healing for both of us. In each case I examined my intent behind wanting to share it. If my intent was for healing and not dumping my stuff on someone else, or if I felt it would not be harmful to the other person to share it, then I did. Otherwise I did my own ceremonies to release it. Sometimes that took the form of writing a letter and then burning it. Other times I took my cares to the ocean and symbolically released them by picking up a rock to represent them and tossing that rock into the water. Any ceremony that represents release helped to take it energetically from my body. Then it was important to replace what I released with loving affirmations of the Truth.

Once I forgave others, I began the work of forgiving myself. I held lots of self-blame for the dysfunction in my family growing up and for things I did that I was not really proud of. It was time to let myself off the hook and to see the innocence in me as well. The ultimate goal for me is to reach the point where I understand there is really nothing to forgive. We all do the best we can with the knowledge we have, and we are all innocent at our core.

Surrender - Letting Go of Our Story

My first conscious experience of surrender was during my healing journey through breast cancer. In the moment when I was standing in the shower crying and asking God to do whatever was best for my children, I knew this was one situation I would not be able to control. The total release of control freed up space for surrender. A relaxing into, and releasing resistance to, what is. A letting go and opening into pure beingness. Surrender was a state of being in my soul, only available in the absence of my body's doing. In that moment I understood I had both seen and unseen support all around me. I did not know what the outcome would be, but I knew there was a bigger plan for my family than I was aware of. Surrendering to that plan, without knowing its details, brought with it the willingness to flow with life.

One of the biggest things I needed to surrender was my attachment to the story of my life. My story was my interpretation of my life, from the child part of me that experienced it. The little girl within me was pretty sure she was right. The challenge was that, from my perceptions, I developed mistaken beliefs about myself. I wondered if it was possible to find another way to look at things. In a way, my brother was right when he said I was causing my own problems. By continuing to hang onto those mistaken beliefs, I was limiting my experience. As I began to tell myself and others a different story, I brought different results energetically. I do matter; I am lovable; I am surrounded by loving beings always; I have value simply by being; and the Universe is a friendly place. Those were some of the Truths I chose as my new story-line.

I demonstrated my new story by my thoughts, words, and actions. I stopped casting villains and victims in the scenarios, and I began to approach things from a perspective of love and respect for all of the many souls who have been my teachers and students in this lifetime.

Surrender allows me to feel the support and connection with the Divine. As I sink into it, I feel total acceptance and infinite love. As I let my illusions of control go, I make space for something new and exciting to take its place.

Trust

The dictionary definition of trust talks about it being a basis of assured or confident reliance on the integrity, strength, ability, surety, etc. of a person or thing. My childhood showed me that the adults, whose job it was to protect me, were the ones who abused me. There were so many lies and so much deception that it was hard to discern the truth, so my level of trust was almost nonexistent. My father once said, "Don't believe anything you hear and only half of what you see." As a young girl I interpreted that to mean I should not trust anyone or anything. Today, I do not think that was exactly what he meant, but I never asked him for an explanation then. I carried that perception with me until I was 35.

Trust was something I began to experience through the connection my mother and I started to build in the last year of her life. When my mother and I were both in that vulnerable state of a health crisis, we were able to meet each other from the love that was at the core of us all along. There was no time for games or pretence. We said what we meant, and meant what we said. Those honest interactions from our hearts opened up a window for us both.

I trusted in myself at a certain level for most of my life because I thought I was the one who looked after me. I developed a very good built-in warning system in the form of my intuition that guided me. Trust in others began to build slowly in my mom's last days. Trust in God/Goddess developed more slowly. Gradually all three pieces came together and my trust expanded to an understanding that I can handle anything in my life because I do not have to rely solely on my own resources. I am not alone.

I now believe my father's quote was referring to how perception can distort things. I think he was talking about tapping into both our inner resources and Spirit to discern the Truth.

Faith

Where trust for me was more about a belief in someone or something visible, faith was a confident expectation of future events or outcomes. Of things not seen: hope, so to speak. This was a concept that was relatively new to me. My past conditioning prepared me to expect the worst and to be pleasantly surprised if the worst did not happen. Faith was asking me to choose another way of approaching things.

The kind of faith I am referring to differs from the concept of faith that is prevalent in some religious traditions, where there is some all-seeing all-knowing presence, separate from us, that we hand our accountability over to. I am not interested in any dogma that supports separation and exclusion, or promotes a right way or a wrong way of communing with the God of your understanding. There are as many paths to rediscovering the Divinity within you as there are people. I love Rumi's quote, "Beyond our ideas of right-doing and wrong-doing, there is a field. I'll meet you there."

Faith, for me, is a deep inner knowing that I am not alone, the Universe is friendly, I am an equal part of a larger whole, and all events in my life are being orchestrated for my highest good. Being part of that larger whole does not include a better than/less than kind of relationship with anyone or anything. It is an equal relationship of power with everyone and everything. God/Goddess is not something external. It is a part of me, as I am a part of it. From this perspective of power with, all things are possible.

With this type of faith, my outward experience does not have to change for my inner experience to change. I symbolically sing my heart song, even if I cannot imagine who would want to hear it. It is the song I was born to sing, and no one else can sing it the way I can. In the singing of it I become the conduit for Spirit. The thought that I am an equal part in a larger whole, together with the feeling of hope, brings forth inspired creations through me.

Faith and hope have been whispering to me all my life. I now listen to the whispers. I believe in my dreams, because I know they have been Divinely delivered to me. My choice is in whether or not I accept Spirit's invitation to be a channel for them. Living my dreams in no way detracts from anyone else living theirs. We are co-creating in an abundant Universe where there is more than enough for all of us.

The Web of Life

There really is no question in my heart anymore about whether or not we are all connected. The question I continue to ask myself is, "What am I doing, or not doing, that sometimes blocks the experience of connection?" When I get out of my head and allow myself to get down to a heart level with people, I experience oneness. In those moments of vulnerability, I am able to see beyond the surface differences and find our common humanity.

I think it is time to open the eyes of our hearts and take a good look around. Every one of our thoughts, words, and actions affects us and others. There are no exceptions to this. We live on a diverse planet of global interdependence between people, places, and things. We need to respect and appreciate them all. Somewhere along the line, humans came up with the mistaken premise they were independent and superior. This division is evident between humans and other living organisms, and sadly it is most evident in human relationships between races, cultures, religions, and genders. This has led us on a potentially disastrous course. We are killing each other and the planet at an alarming rate.

The good news is we are all powerful creators. Because we are interconnected, as each one of us does our work to experience more moments of peace in our daily lives, we shift our consciousness. As we do the work to heal our past on an individual level, we will also impact consciousness on a global level. Together we can recreate an extraordinary world.

Honouring Our Ancestors

I come from a long line of courageous women and men who did their best. My mother loved me, even if she could not love me in the way I wanted to be loved. She was not able to see my pain because she had not dealt with her own. My father doted on me in the short time he was physically present in my life. He departed way sooner than I would have liked, but he left me with a deep appreciation for the gift of life.

I miss the physical presence of both of my parents. I keep them with me always by embodying all they taught me and sharing it with others. I do this by carrying forward their traits that make for a more loving world and leaving the rest behind. I bless all of my ancestors with unconditional love and deep gratitude for all they did to pave the way and make it possible for me to be the best person I can be. Without them I would not be here. I respect their wisdom and their ingenuity.

I believe I chose both of my parents, before my soul incarnated into my physical body, so I could experience all I have experienced in order to be able to teach others from that place. I teach some of the things they forgot about love and life, and I would not have known to teach them without having experienced their absence. I no longer blame them for any of my shortcomings. The degree to which my behaviour is a cry for love is equivalent to the depth of my inner pain, in the same way as it was for my ancestors. My behaviour belongs to me, and I am accountable for cleaning it up. The only person's behaviour I can truly change is my own.

The greatest way I know to honour myself, my ancestors, and the generations that will come after me is to do my own healing work to stop dysfunction from being passed down through the generations. The impact of that goes far beyond what the eye can see. There are some Native cultures that believe the healing travels energetically seven generations forward and seven generations back. I love that visual, and I choose to believe it too. I am humbled by the possibilities inherent in each of us cleaning up our own past, our little pieces of the Universe.

To my mother and father and all the women and men in my family system who have come before me, I love you and I thank you from the bottom of my heart for all that you gave and all that you could not give. I honour all of your sacrifices and I grieve your losses. I carry your innocence, your Divinity, and your courage with me in my body, mind, emotions, and spirit. Thank you for being with me all ways and for holding space from beyond the veil so that my daughters and I can continue to find strength in forgiveness, surrender, trust, faith, and vulnerability. May my generation and your grandchildren's be the ones to find and use our voices to freely express our magnificence to the world. As women, may we learn to cultivate healthy, inclusive, compassionate, and spiritual relationships with men. Thank you for helping us to welcome those men into our lives with respect. Please guide them to their hearts so they can treat the women in their lives with reverence. Let us all go home together.

And so it is.

Going Home Together

Here we are at the end of this part of our journey together. I am deeply honoured you have chosen to accompany me through the pages of this book, and that you have been a witness to my life. I hope in some small way you have found sameness, connection, comfort, reassurance, and peace here. Most of all, I hope that you have found love. Love of Self, love of other, and the love of your Creator. You are a child of God/Goddess and so deserving of that love.

When I began this book I had no idea how profoundly I would be impacted by the writing of it. What started out as a process of recording some of the events of my life, with the intent to help others heal, turned into a generational love story. *ACIM* talks about miracles being a shift in perception from fear to love. In that context, writing this book was a miracle. Healing occurred for me, at a deeper level than it ever had before, as I revisited my past with new eyes. Through honouring the experiences of my family, I saw how love was waiting patiently for me to claim it all the time. From being reunited with my mom before her death, to my mom and dad being reunited in death, to me being reunited energetically with my ancestors through something as simple as researching my genealogy, I was able to move from anger to forgiveness. And beyond that to an experience of gratitude and grace. I transcended the sadness and the pain of my past and learned to fly. Contrary to my expectations, it was not a solo flight. I carry my ancestors' wisdom and experience on my wings energetically, no longer with the heavy energy of fear and blame, but rather with the lightness of love and innocence.

The most critical piece in my healing so far has been the process of forgiving, letting go, and restoring the relationship with my own mother. I have learned to shed the tears my foremothers were not able to shed and process the grief for the women from current and previous generations. In so doing, I believe I am shifting my family's emotional patterns and handing down a different model of creative health to my daughters. As far as the relationship with my father goes, I feel he and I are still working on a few more healing pieces between us. I cannot tell you at this point exactly what they are, but my intuition tells me we are not yet complete. I have faith we will resolve what needs to be resolved, and I am open to his help in doing that. My intent is that the potential for self-healing becomes the new legacy in my family system.

You may wonder where I am now on my journey. The ego part of me would like to be able to tell you I am living peacefully and authentically 100 percent of the time. But the truth is I am human and sometimes catch myself reverting back to my old patterns of sleep-walking through life. Thankfully, I do not usually remain in that state for long. Inevitably the Universe will deliver a sign to me that will wake me up again and remind me how much I value consciousness. Living in peace, joy, and love are my preferences. The more I walk my own talk, the closer I am to those states of being. I am continually moving towards the next highest version of who I am and I am definitely a work in progress.

I have become more of my authentic Self though. The prospect of dying stripped away all my layers of pretence and social convention. The masks I wore to please others dangle lifelessly now, rendered useless in the face of Real Life. I learned what Real Life meant to me. Real Life is not about *doing*. It is about continuing to uncover who the Real Me is, and then *being* that person everywhere I am. Real Life is about relationships: the one I have with my Self, the ones I have with others, and the one I have transpersonally with the world and my Creator, discovering my greater purpose for being here.

I am no longer defined by the roles I took on to survive my childhood. I am now a Divine expression of mother energy, instead of a caretaker. I am able to hold the space for others to find their own way, no longer acting as a saviour. I am blessed with the wisdom passed down through the ages and able to offer that gift to others unconditionally, rather than playing the role of the smart one. I am connected to a vast network of spiritual energy working together for a Divine purpose, and I am not the one in control trying to hold it all together anymore. From this place, what comes through me are acts of pure love.

My past experiences prepared me to be in service to the world as a teacher and a mentor, to extend compassion, nonjudgement, and love in all circumstances. It has taught me about the embodiment of true feminine strength: not power over, but the authentic power of standing for who I am. Having lived through some very dark times and moved from surviving to thriving, I can inspire and encourage others. I can see into the heart and soul of another. I can meet you where you are and energetically hold space for you to discover your own Truth. I can be the voice for those not yet able to speak. I have learned the Universe is a friendly and a safe place.

This journey has given me a clearer picture of who I am and what I stand for in the world. I stand for love, spirituality, and integrity. I stand for magnitude: not someone else's definition of that word, but my own brand of magnitude, which is quiet, gentle, solid, grounded, and connected to Source. I stand for authentic power: power with, not power over. I stand for allowing myself to dream and following those dreams, no matter what. I stand for being authentic in all of my relationships and showing the Real Me, not just the parts I think will be accepted. I stand for social and spiritual inclusion. I stand for believing in and teaching others that it matters we are here, and that we all have a unique contribution to the world. I stand for choice.

Who am I really? I am not the roles I play, and I am not broken. I am whole and complete. I do not have to do anything, say anything, or be anything to matter. I am a spirit having a human experience, a Goddess, love embodied, light, and a fellow journeyer finding my way home to my Self. Who I am in this moment is enough. I am a very rich woman in matters of the heart, which is the only thing that really matters. Because we are all interconnected, interrelated, and interdependent, you are these things too. We are all going home together.

You do not have to do anything to be accepted and loved because you *are* love. You are worthy and you matter because you Are. My hope is that you will make this book a celebration of your own journey of bringing all the parts of you home. That you will find peace in your heart. You are not alone. We all need to be the peace we want to see in the world, and peace begins with you and me. It is not a by-product of 'doing'. Peace is the result of being fully present in every moment.

I feel blessed to be on this path of discovery with all of you. At this point in my life there are two things I know for sure. One is that there are no mistakes in the Universe. There is a reason you found your way to this book. My hope is that it invites you into the realm of possibility.

The other thing I am certain of is that our lives are sacred paths with value and purpose. Every one of us is pure love and an incredible physical manifestation of the Divine. There are no exceptions to this. This is the Truth about you. Cast anything that does not reflect this out of your mind and heart.

Stand with me in your Truth for a moment and breathe it in. Feel the remembrance of it beginning to illuminate every cell in your body. I ask you to consider shining this light, in your own unique way, every day of your life. The world will be a better place for your having done so.

The door to infinite hope, love, and possibility is always open. Spirit is calling you to something bigger, and you already have all of the resources within you to facilitate that journey. I will be walking beside you energetically, with love, as you step over the threshold of the old to embrace the extraordinary life that awaits you. As you come back to your heart, in the recognition of the Divinity within you, you will find your way back to your Self. Welcome home!

Tools for Transformation

- *Practise the four cornerstones of peace: forgiveness, surrender, trust and faith.*

- *Write a letter to your ancestors thanking them for the gift of life.*

- *Be your Self and allow your magnificence to light up the world.*

Conclusion: The Fairy Tale Revisited - Life beyond the Wall

The Conclusion of the Fairy Tale from the Prologue, Told from the Perspective of Love, Where Our True Selves Are Honoured and Hope Is Embraced

AS SHE BEGAN TO LET HER REAL SELF PEEK out between the cracks in the mortar, the princess discovered there was a whole other world beyond the Kingdom she knew. She caught sight of the Kingdom of Nothing Real Can Be Threatened in the distance. This was a world that knew the Truth of who she really was. It appeared to be within her reach. To travel to the new Kingdom though, the princess knew she would have to leave behind her marriage, and she let that fear keep her imprisoned for a while longer.

Then one day she finally realised that, to remain in the Kingdom of Smoke and Mirrors with the prince, she would have to sell her soul. Ultimately she knew at the core of her being that was too high a price to pay. She found the only way she could have access to the new Kingdom was to begin to take down the wall around her heart. As she removed each brick from the wall she could see more and more of the Kingdom of Nothing Real Can Be Threatened. She began to recover her buried Self.

The princess began with the 'GROW UP: BE AN ADULT' layer. To her amazement, as each brick was cast aside she uncovered the innocent child within her. This was the part of her that knew creativity and spontaneity and freedom and that it was okay to play and have fun. Wonder and magic began to come back into her life.

The next layer to come down was 'DO NOT EVER FAIL'. Once the princess realised that there was no such thing as failure, she could choose to look at things that did not go according to plan as signposts

231

pointing her in a new direction. They became stepping stones to something even better. Free of the shackles of this layer the princess could now scale the wall and began to venture more and more into the unknown. She met new people and tried new things. Contrary to her fear of not getting another chance to win the queen's love or losing the king's adoration, she discovered her worth was not determined by what she did. She was lovable and adorable just by being. She had no control over what others thought of her. The only thing she had control of was her own thoughts and actions.

Then she came to the 'STOP FEELING' layer. To remove these bricks meant the princess would need to feel all those feelings she had avoided since she was a little girl. Whether they had been stuffed down with food or sidestepped by leaving her body energetically, this part of the journey required that she get in touch with her body and listen to its wisdom. The feelings did not destroy her or engulf her as she feared. Feeling them lifted the heavy cloak that had been covering up her joy. She learned all of her feelings were okay and if she stayed with them she could ride their ebb and flow through the current of her life. She could be the witness to her own process and then make a decision about how, or even if, she needed to respond to them. Each brick in this layer held a key to unlock her past.

With three of the four layers of bricks removed the new kingdom was becoming more and more her reality. All that remained was the 'BE QUIET' layer. This final row had been in place the longest and required some serious work to dislodge. To remove it meant not only finding her voice but then also having the courage to use it wherever and whenever she was called to learn and to teach. To move beyond this roadblock the princess needed to believe she mattered and that her life had meaning and purpose. When the final layer was dismantled she began to sing from the rooftops. Then on other days she was quiet. She now knew she had a choice.

Along the way some of the bricks were more challenging to remove than others, but she found if she asked for help the load was lightened.

She found that on the darkest days, if she was able to open up her heart and receive the unconditional love she so willingly shared with others, she was surrounded by earth angels who gave her wings and showed her how to fly.

As the princess allowed herself to set down the baggage from her past, she freed herself and her ancestors. She taught her children it was okay to do the same. She is still a work in progress, but she soars with the eagles now, forever grateful for a friendly Universe and joyful with each opportunity for personal growth on her journey home.

She lives peacefully ever after.

Conclusion

Resources

SELF-LOVE MEDITATION

GET COMFORTABLE IN YOUR CHAIR. Put your feet flat on the floor. Close your eyes and begin to relax. Take three deep breaths in and let them out with a sigh. You do not have to do or be anything in this place. Let go of anything that may be weighing heavy on your heart. Your guides and angels will hold all of that for you. Just let it go. Feel the weight of your body in the chair and notice the way the chair is supporting you. Notice how effortlessly your breath comes into your body and then goes out. Feel the rhythm of your chest rising and falling with each breath.

I would like you to imagine you are a tree and that there are roots extending from the bottoms of your feet. Those roots go down deep into the centre of the earth and are anchoring you securely. Feel their strength and how they are grounding you in place. As you take a breath in, imagine drawing up energy from the centre of Mother Earth. This energy is a deep rich shade of brown. Feel it moving up through your feet. Keep breathing and slowly drawing the energy up through your body. As it moves up your legs the colour is shifting to a beautiful deep shade of red. Now it has reached the bottom of your spine and is beginning to slowly move up through the middle of your body. As it passes your abdomen the colour is shifting to a vibrant orange, and then a brilliant yellow as it moves up from your belly button. You have now drawn the energy all the way up to the centre of your heart and the colour has shifted to an emerald green. Continue breathing, imagining that beautiful emerald green colour and feeling the love from Mother Earth in the centre of your heart. Let your heart hold that energy.

On an in breath, imagine drawing energy down from Father Sky. It is a beautiful ray of iridescent white and gold light. As you continue breathing imagine that energy entering your body through the top of your head. The colour begins to turn into a beautiful vibrant shade of violet. And now it is moving down past the middle of your forehead and changing to purple. As it continues down your body towards your throat the colour is shifting to blue. Slowly, as you continue to breathe, the blue energy moves toward your heart centre and blends with the emerald green that is already there. Feel how you are a perfect, balanced blend of earth and sky. Now breathe into that green in your heart centre and allow it to expand. And as you breathe out, imagine that healing, loving, peaceful emerald green extending out around you. With each out breath it extends further and further. It fills the room. And then it fills the neighbourhood. It keeps extending further and further. Now it fills the city. Then the country and the rest of the planet. Notice how powerful you are in this inner place of love and peace.

And now I would like you to take a deep breath in and slowly begin to bring that emerald green energy back to the centre of your heart. Place your hands over your heart. From this place you are going to extend that love to all the parts of your body. Start by moving your hands to the top of your head and send love to your amazing brain. Thank it for the thousands of things it does for you every minute of every day. It never stops trying to look after you and keep all the parts of your body working in synch. Then move your hands over your eyes. Send them love and thank them for their gift of sight. Then put your hands over your ears and thank them for the gift of hearing. Touch your nose and send it gratitude for taking in the breath of life and for your sense of smell. Then on to your mouth. Touch your lips and send them gratitude for the gift of taste and speech and their ability to kiss the ones you love. Now we are moving down to your throat. Place your hands on or near your throat. Send it loving energy for its help in delivering nutrition to your body and extending your voice out into the world. Move your hands down the front of your body. Touch your breasts and send loving energy to them. They serve so many purposes. Perhaps they have nursed a child or been a source of sexual pleasure. Thank them for their beauty, no matter what their shape or size. And thank them for their sensitivity. Move your hands down to your stomach. What a marvel your stomach is. It is a safe container for so many of the organs that sustain your life. It expands and contracts with each breath. It is your soft centre of vulnerability. It feels the pulse of life and sends and receives energetic messages for you. Send it loving blessings. Now place your hands on your thighs and send loving energy to your legs and feet. They carry you through the world and help you keep your balance. Bring your attention to your arms. Place each hand on the top of the opposite arm. Send your arms loving energy through your hands and thank them for the hundreds of tasks they help you with every day. With your arms crossed reach your hands towards your back, giving yourself a hug. Imagine your body bathed in the warmth of that beautiful emerald green light. If there is any part of you that might be out of alignment with Source at the moment, send an extra burst of light to that part. Feel in every cell of your body what an incredible being of light you are. Thank your body for the magnificent creation that it is. It is the vehicle that carries you through life. Thank your guides and angels for being with you. Not only during this meditation, but each and every day. And thank yourself for your willingness to go on this journey.

With your eyes still closed I want you to begin to bring yourself back into the room. Take three deep breaths in and out. Feel yourself in your body and feel the chair underneath you. Begin to wiggle your fingers and your toes. Feel your feet on the floor. And when you are ready open your eyes and come back into the room.

Namasté

VALUES LIST

acceptance

achievement

aesthetics

assertiveness

career/work

caring

challenge

comfort

commitment

compassion

consciousness

co-operation

courage

courtesy

creativity

diligence

diversity

education

emotional well-being

empathy

equality

faith

family

financial security

financial serenity

flexibility

forgiveness

freedom

generosity

gentleness

gratitude

harmony

health

helpfulness

heritage

hobbies

honesty

honour

humility

independence

integrity

joy

justice

kindness

love

loyalty

mental well-being

openness

orderliness

parenthood

patience

peace

personal growth

personal power

physical well-being

pleasure

power

prestige

privacy

purpose

quality marriage

quality relationships

recognition

reliability

respect

responsibility

self-discipline

service

sexual fulfillment

spiritual well-being

sports

success

tolerance

trust

uniqueness

unity

FEELINGS LIST

abandoned
able to cope
abusive
accepted
accepting
adept
adequate
affectionate
afraid
aggravated
aggressive
agitated
agonised
agreeable
alive
alone
amazed
ambivalent
amused
angry
animated
annoyed
anxious
apathetic
apologetic
appreciated
appreciative
arrogant
ashamed
astonished
attached
attentive
attractive
authentic
bad
baffled

balanced
beautiful
betrayed
bewildered
bitchy
bitter
blissful
bold
bored
bothered
brave
bubbly
burned out
callous
calm
cantankerous
capable
captivated
cared for
carefree
caring
cautious
cheerful
child-like
clear
closed
cold
comfortable
committed
compassionate
competent
composed
concerned
confident
confused
congruent

connected
conscious
considerate
considered
content(ed)
controlled
controlling
cornered
courageous
cosy
crazy
creative
critical
criticised
crushed
curious
defeated
defenseless
defensive
dejected
delighted
delirious
depressed
deserving
desirable
despairing
detached
determined
devastated
devoted
different
disappointed
disapproving
disbelieving
disconnected
discounted

discouraged	fidgety	helpless
disgusted	flabbergasted	hesitant
disinterested	flat	hopeful
displeased	flattered	hopeless
disrespected	flustered	horrible
distressed	foolish	horrified
disturbed	forgiving	hospitable
doubtful	forgotten	hostile
driven	forlorn	humiliated
dubious	fortunate	hurried
eager	fragile	hurt
ecstatic	frail	hysterical
edgy	frantic	ignored
elated	free	ill at ease
embarrassed	friendly	immobilised
emotional	frightened	immoral
empathetic	frozen	impatient
emphatic	frustrated	impetuous
empty	fulfilled	important
enamoured	fuming	imposed upon
enchanted	furious	impressed
energetic	generous	in the way
enjoyment	gentle	inadequate
enlightened	giddy	incensed
enraged	glad	included
enriched	glum	indifferent
enthusiastic	good	inferior
envious	gracious	infuriated
euphoric	grateful	inhibited
exasperated	great	innocent
excited	gregarious	insecure
exhausted	grieving	intelligent
expressive	grouchy	interested
failure	guilty	intimidated
fantastic	happy	invigorated
fascinated	harassed	involved
fearful	hated	irrational
fed up	hateful	irritable
feeble	healthy	irritated
feminine	helpful	jealous

joyful	out of control	regretful
judged	outgoing	rejected
judgemental	outraged	relaxed
kind	overjoyed	relieved
lazy	overwhelmed	repelled
left out	overworked	repulsed
let down	pained	resentful
lively	panicky	resigned
lonely	paralysed	respectful
looked up to	paranoid	responsible
lost	passionate	responsive
loved	passive	restful
lovestruck	patient	restless
loving	peaceful	restrained
lucky	pensive	revengeful
mad	perplexed	revitalised
manipulated	perturbed	ridiculous
marvelous	pessimistic	rigid
masculine	placated	romantic
masterful	playful	sad
mean	pleased	safe
meddlesome	positive	satisfied
meditative	possessive	scared
melancholic	powerful	secure
mischievous	powerless	seductive
miserable	pressured	seething
morose	productive	sensitive
mortified	prosperous	sentimental
mixed up	protective	separate
mystified	proud	serene
needed	purposeful	sexy
needy	put down	shaken
negative	put upon	shaky
neglected	puzzled	shamed
nervous	qualified	shocked
numb	quiet	shy
obstinate	rational	sick
offended	real	sincere
open	receptive	skeptical
optimistic	refreshed	small

smug	threatened	unwelcome
sociable	thrilled	unworthy
solemn	tired	uplifted
sorry	tolerant	upset
spontaneous	tormented	uptight
stifled	tortured	used
stimulated	tough	useless
strong	tranquil	valued
stubborn	trapped	vibrant
stumped	triumphant	victorious
stunned	troubled	violated
stupid	trusted	virile
subdued	trusting	vivacious
submissive	ugly	vulnerable
successful	uncared for	wanted
supported	uncertain	warm-hearted
sure	uncomfortable	wary
surly	unconcerned	weak
surprised	undecided	weary
suspicious	understood	whole
sympathetic	uneasy	wild
tactful	unfeeling	withdrawn
talented	unhappy	wonderful
tender(ness)	uninhibited	worried
tense	unloved	worthless
terrified	unreasonable	worthy
thankful	unsure	
thoughtful	unwanted	

MY PERSONAL RESOURCE LIST

A Course in Miracles, Foundation for Inner Peace

Agnew, Eleanor and Robideaux, Sharon, *My Mama's Waltz: A Book for Daughters of Alcoholic Mothers*

Ban Breathnach, Sarah, *Simple Abundance: A Daybook of Comfort and Joy*, www.simpleabundance.com

Beattie, Melody, *Codependent No More: How to Stop Controlling Others and Start Caring for Yourself*, www.melodybeattie.com

Beck, Martha, *Finding Your Own North Star: Claiming the Life You Were Meant to Live*, www.marthabeck.com

Berger, Janice, *Emotional Fitness: Discovering Our Natural Healing Power*, www.janiceberger.com

Bradshaw, John, *Homecoming: Reclaiming and Championing Your Inner Child*, www.johnbradshaw.com

Brown, Michael, *The Presence Process*, www.thepresenceportal.com

Cirocco, Grace, *Take the Step and the Bridge Will Be There: Inspiration and Guidance for Moving Your Life Forward*, www.gracecirocco.com

Clearmind International Institute. Professional counsellor training and personal development programs and workshops. www.clearmind.com

Cohen, Alan, *A Deep Breath of Life: Daily Inspiration for Heart-Centered Living*, www.alancohen.com

Dyer, Dr. Wayne W., *The Power of Intention: Learning to Co-create Your World Your Way*, www.drwaynedyer.com

Ehl, Dr. Kevin, Café of Life Chiropractic, Port Moody, British Columbia, Canada. Serving a chiropractic experience that nurtures body, mind, emotions, and spirit. www.cafeportmoody.com

Enya, all of her music soothes my soul. www.enya.com

Fields, David and Faye, *The Invisible Wedding: Exploring the Essence of Spiritual Partnership*, www.theinvisiblewedding.com

Ford, Debbie, *Spiritual Divorce*, www.debbieford.com

Frankl, Viktor E., *Man's Search for Meaning*

Gilbert, Elizabeth, *Eat, Pray, Love: One Woman's Search for Everything Across Italy, India and Indonesia*, www.elizabethgilbert.com

Hagan, Denise. A beautiful Celtic Goddess of story and song. Denise channels God/Goddess in her music and reminds me of the deeper meaning of life always. www.denisehagan.com

Hay, Louise L., *You Can Heal Your Life*, www.louisehay.com

Hendricks Ph.D., Kathlyn & Gay, *The Conscious Heart: Seven Soul Choices That Create Your Relationship Destiny*, www.hendricks.com

Hicks, Esther and Jerry, *The Vortex: Where the Law of Attraction Assembles All Cooperative Relationships*: www.abraham-hicks.com

Jeffers Ph.D., Susan, *Feel the Fear and Do It Anyway*, www.susanjeffers.com

Katie, Byron with Mitchell, Stephen, *Loving What Is: Four Questions that Can Change Your Life*, www.thework.com

Macy, Joanna & Young Brown, Molly, *Coming Back to Life: Practices to Reconnect Our Lives, Our World*

Maté M.D., Gabor, *When The Body Says No: The Cost of Hidden Stress*, www.drgabormate.com

Morrow Lindbergh, Anne, *Gift from the Sea*

Mountain Dreamer, Oriah, *What We Ache For: Creativity and the Unfolding of Your Soul*, www.oriahmountaindreamer.com

Northrup M.D., Christiane, *Mother-Daughter Wisdom: Creating a Legacy of Physical and Emotional Health*, www.drnorthrup.com

O'Donohue, John, *Anam Cara: A Book of Celtic Wisdom*

Pert Ph.D., Candace B., *Molecules of Emotion: The Science Behind Mind-Body Medicine*, www.candacepert.com

Pinkola Estés Ph.D., Clarissa, *Women Who Run with the Wolves*

Richo, David, *How to Be an Adult in Relationships*, www.davericho.com

Roth, Geneen, *Women Food and God: An Unexpected Path to Almost Everything*, www.geneenroth.com

Schwarz, Joyce, *The Vision Board: The Secret to an Extraordinary Life*, www.ihaveavision.org

Siegel, Dr. Bernie S., *Love, Medicine & Miracles*, www.berniesiegelmd.com

Steinem, Gloria, *Revolution from Within: A Book of Self-Esteem*, www.gloriasteinem.com

Tolle, Eckhart, *A New Earth: Awakening to Your Life's Purpose*, www.eckharttolle.com

Vanzant, Iyanla, *One Day My Soul Just Opened Up: 40 Days and 40 Nights Toward Spiritual Strength and Personal Growth*, www.innervisionsworldwide.com

Viorst, Judith, *Necessary Losses*

Walsch, Neale Donald, *Conversations With God* series, www.nealedonaldwalsch.com

Whyte, David, *The Heart Aroused: Poetry and the Preservation of the Soul in Corporate America*, www.davidwhyte.com

Williamson, Marianne, *A Return To Love*, www.marianne.com

Zukav, Gary, *The Seat of the Soul*, www.zukav.com

About The Author

Denise Cunningham holds a BA in transpersonal counselling psychology, and is a Registered Professional Counsellor with the Canadian Professional Counsellors Association. She is also an inspirational speaker, Reiki Master, ThetaHealing™ practitioner, Quantum Touch practitioner, spiritual healer, sacred group/retreat facilitator, and an intuitive fabric artist. Her career in the healing arts has spanned two decades, and her journey through a life threatening illness provided her with a renewed perspective on living that she 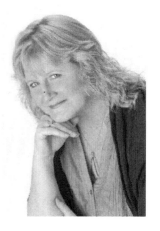 incorporates into her work. She is the mother of two beautiful daughters who are her greatest teachers. In life and in work, Denise leads with her heart in providing a compassionate healing space of safety, acceptance and respect. A living example of not only surviving...but thriving, Denise is passionate about empowering others to do the same.

Dubbed the "Hope Whisperer", Denise is a spiritual visionary who has had the ability to see into the heart and soul of people since she was a little girl. She teaches that there is hope in every situation. Denise holds the sacred Truth she sees in others, and reflects it back to them, until they are able to see it for themselves. This gift has led her on many adventures and has provided lots of material for her writing, workshops, teaching, and speaking engagements. In her down-time she loves to centre herself by spending time in nature. The trees, mountains, and ocean all call to her, so it is not surprising that beautiful British Columbia, Canada has been her home for the past 15 years. Denise also loves to create intuitive fabric art. Something in the way that colour, texture, design and Divine guidance come together in a piece speaks to her soul. Her vision is to co-create a more peaceful, loving, and harmonious world by helping individuals to create more peaceful, loving, and harmonious lives. Denise supports a holistic approach to health.

Next Steps...

Please visit *www.journeyhome.ca* for further information on Denise Cunningham and her spiritual healing practices. There you will find her upcoming workshops, sacred groups/retreats, and examples of her intuitive fabric art. To book Denise for a keynote speech, please contact her at ~~denise@journeyhome.ca.~~ hopewhisperer-777@gmail.com

Journey Home Healing Arts
Fostering Peace & Harmony
In Body, Mind & Spirit

Made in the USA
Charleston, SC
26 May 2012